Metaphorical Signs in Computed Tomography of Chest and Abdomen

Andrey Yudin

Metaphorical Signs in Computed Tomography of Chest and Abdomen

Springer

Andrey Yudin
Department of Radiology
Russian National Research Medical University
Moscow
Russia

The Work was first published in 2012 by Prof. Dr. Andrey Yudin.

ISBN 978-3-319-34965-7 ISBN 978-3-319-04013-4 (eBook)
DOI 10.1007/978-3-319-04013-4
Springer Cham Heidelberg New York Dordrecht London

Softcover reprint of the hardcover 1st edition 2014

Printed on acid-free paper

Springer is part of Springer Science+Business Media (www.springer.com)

From the Author

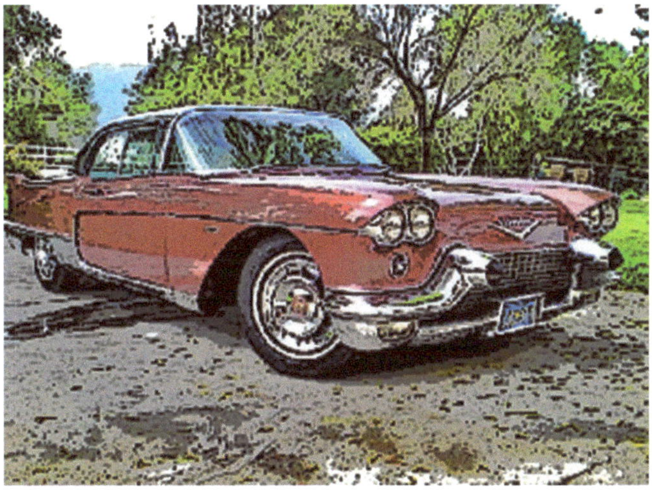

Cadillac Eldorado 1957 *model*.

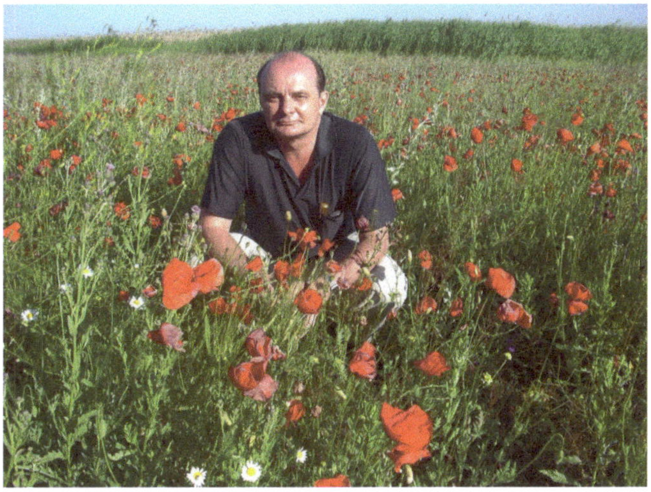

Andrey Yudin was born in 1957.

Much in common: the same age, the exclusive models, all options, in good working conditions, with no rot and rust, sit down and drive, some problems on the body, etc.

… Long ago in some of the radiology papers, I found a discussion concerning the peculiarities of the names of symptoms: if they are given the names of the authors, then we do not understand their meaning (after all, our specialty is largely metaphorical), and if we have a picturesque description of the image, then it is sometimes excessively emotional. As an example of a failed metaphorical formation, they cited the "1957 Cadillac Lights" sign. Not everyone in the world does know about this car; who knows?

However, the well-known saying insists: "If you did one million bucks – buy the pink Cadillac to success unless that luck turns away!"

I hope this publication will help you get lucky in our profession. Enjoy imaginative perception of radiology!

I want to tell the truth which I do not know, but I'm looking for it.

Professor A. Yudin

Contents

Saber-Sheath Trachea

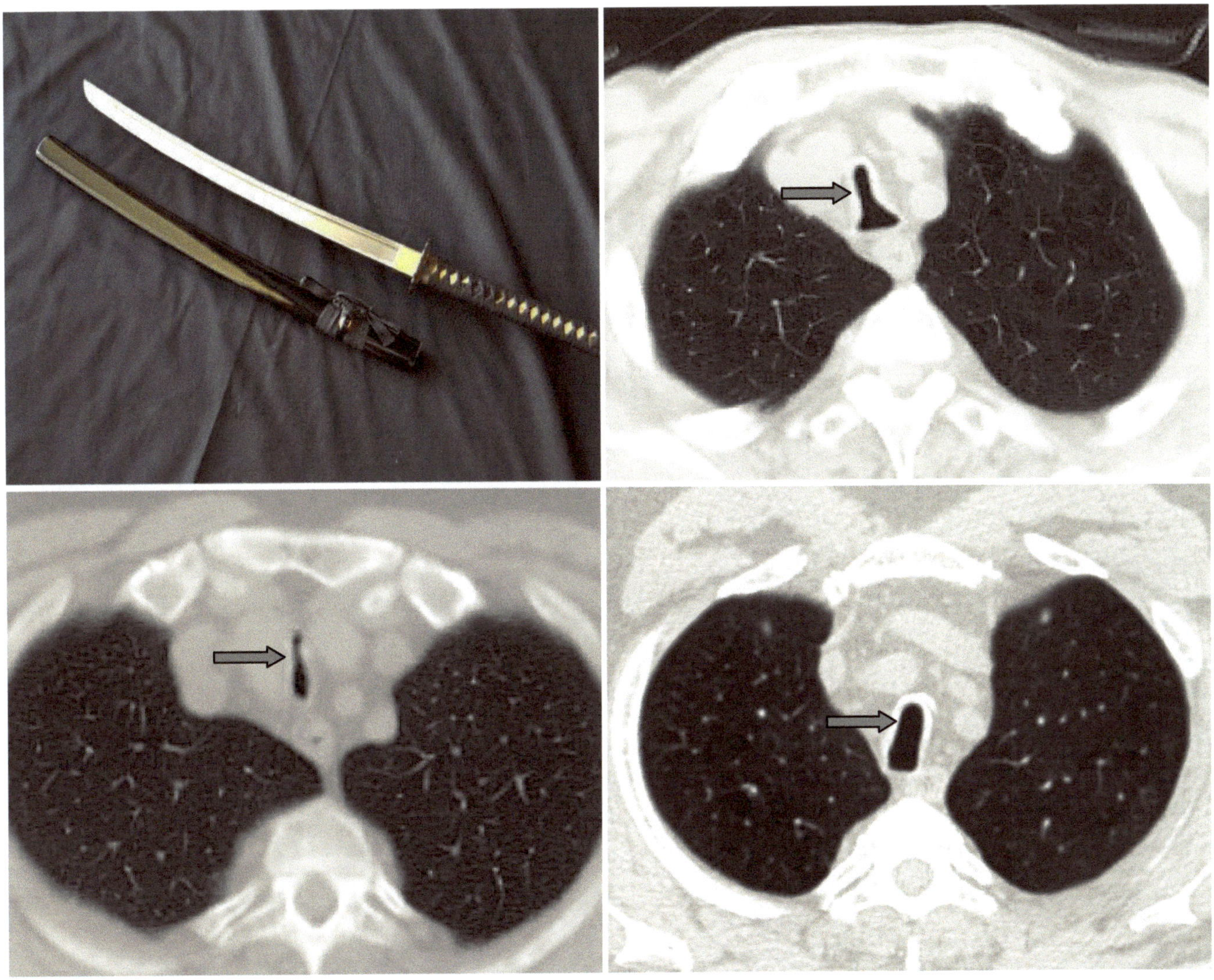

Saber-sheath trachea (↑) refers to diffuse coronal narrowing of the intrathoracic portion of the trachea with concomitant widening of the sagittal diameter. Inward bowing or displacement of the lateral tracheal walls as a result of cartilage weakness is a type of tracheal collapse seen in chronic obstructive pulmonary disease. The sagittal-to-coronal diameter is over 2:1, and the extrathoracic portion of the trachea is not narrowed. Mild intrathoracic tracheal wall thickening and ossifications of tracheal rings can also be seen. There may be further inward bowing of lateral tracheal walls during forceful expiration.

A. Yudin, *Metaphorical Signs in Computed Tomography of Chest and Abdomen*,
DOI 10.1007/978-3-319-04013-4_1, © Springer International Publishing Switzerland 2014

Eggshell Calcification and Rim Enhancement

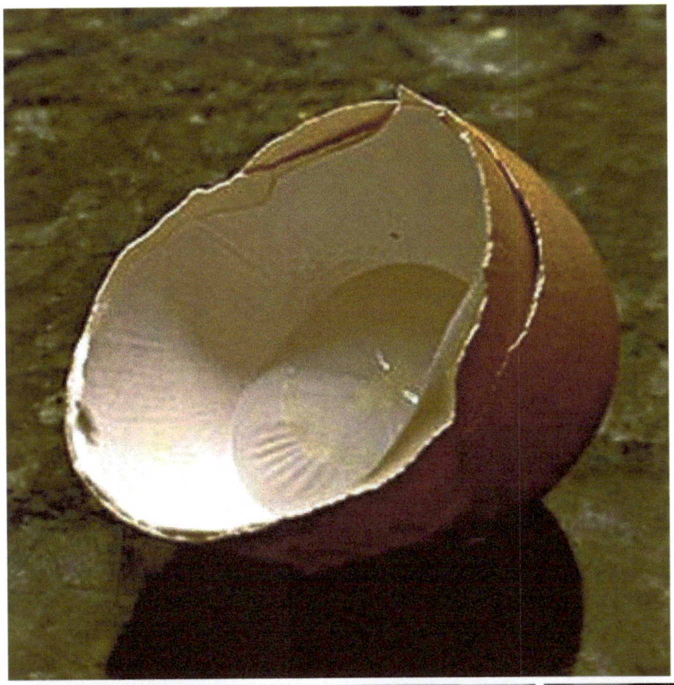

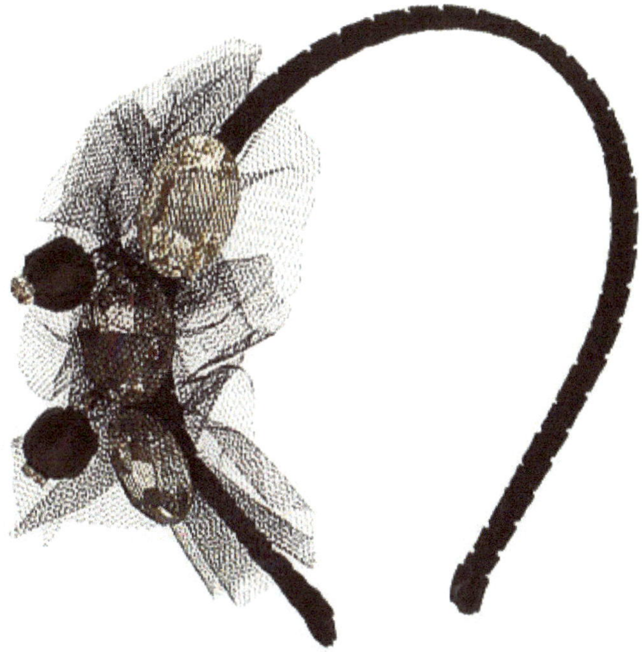

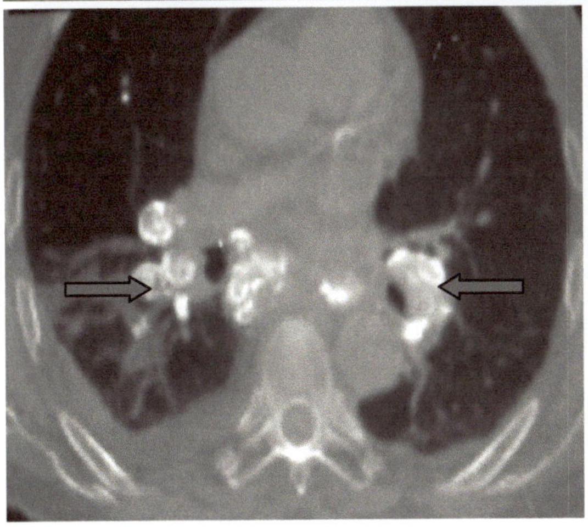

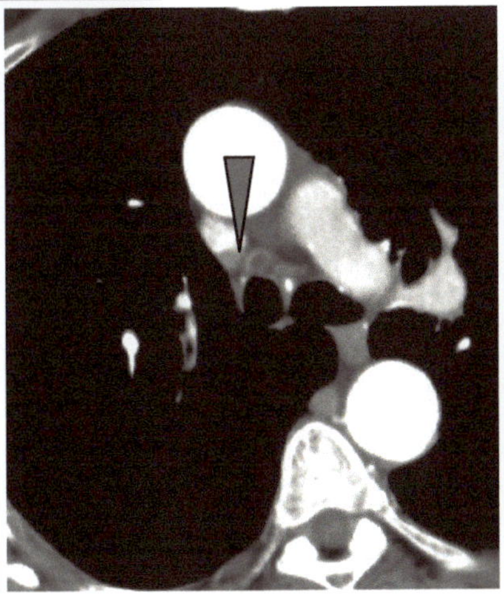

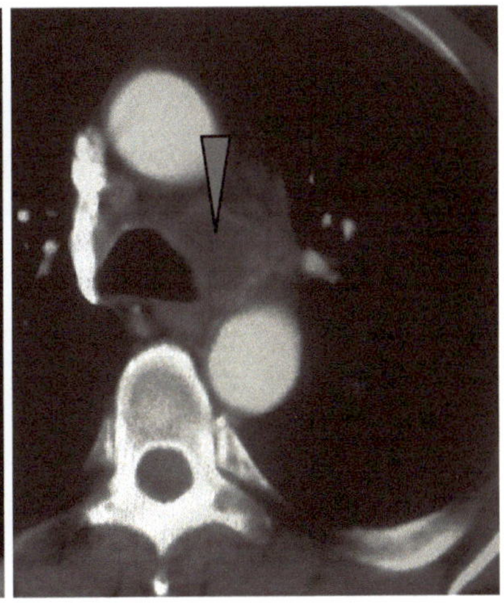

Eggshell calcification (↑) refers to the peripheral rim of calcium deposited in enlarged mediastinal and/or hilar and peribronchial lymph nodes. Shell-like calcifications up to 2 mm thick must be present in at least two lymph nodes; one of the affected lymph nodes must be larger than 1 cm in its greatest diameter. This pattern is most commonly seen in silicosis and coal worker's pneumoconiosis. It may also be seen with sarcoidosis, after radiation therapy to lymph nodes affected by lymphoma, scleroderma, amyloidosis, blastomycosis, and histoplasmosis.

Rim Enhancement (Δ). Necrosis in lymph nodes causes decrease in attenuation within central portions (up to fatty density). This pattern is characteristically associated with mycobacterium infection (tuberculous and nontuberculous). Following contrast administration lymph nodes show peripheral enhancement of capsules. With appropriate clinical data, this pattern may indicate active tuberculosis (or nontuberculous mycobacteria infection) in children and immunocompromised adults.

A. Yudin, *Metaphorical Signs in Computed Tomography of Chest and Abdomen*,
DOI 10.1007/978-3-319-04013-4_2, © Springer International Publishing Switzerland 2014

Split Pleura Sign

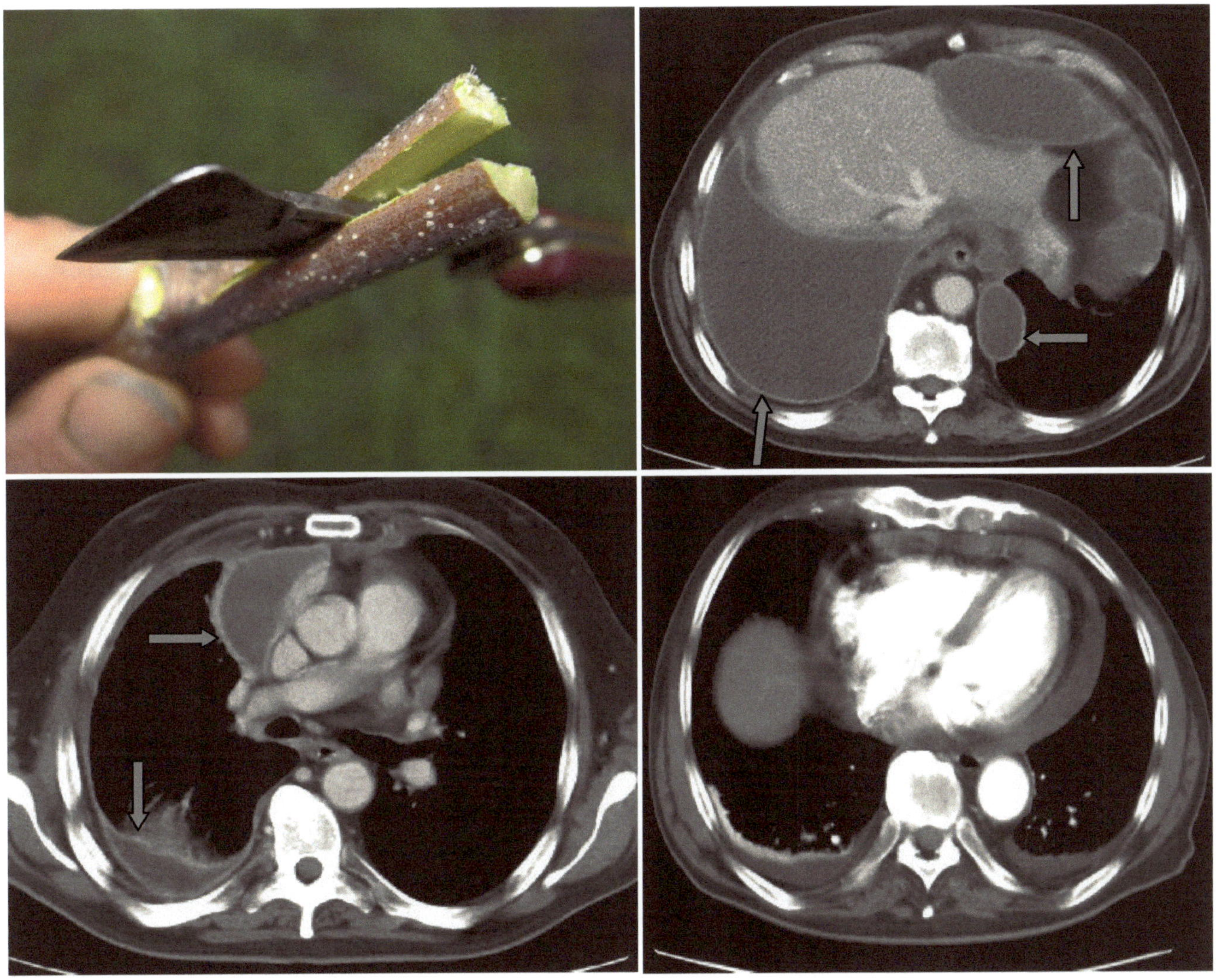

The *split pleura* sign (↑) is seen with pleural empyemas and is considered the most reliable CT sign helping to distinguish empyemas from noninfectious pleural effusions. The sign results from fibrin coating of both the parietal and visceral surface of the pleura with resulting ingrowth of blood vessels. Following IV contrast injection CT shows a loculated fluid collection and thickened pleural layers with accompanying enhancement. Both layers of the pleura can then be visualized as linear regions of enhancement that divide around a less dense empyema or in other words come together at the margins of the collection. Do not confuse with subpleural lung consolidation (image right below).

A. Yudin, *Metaphorical Signs in Computed Tomography of Chest and Abdomen*,
DOI 10.1007/978-3-319-04013-4_3,

Consolidation

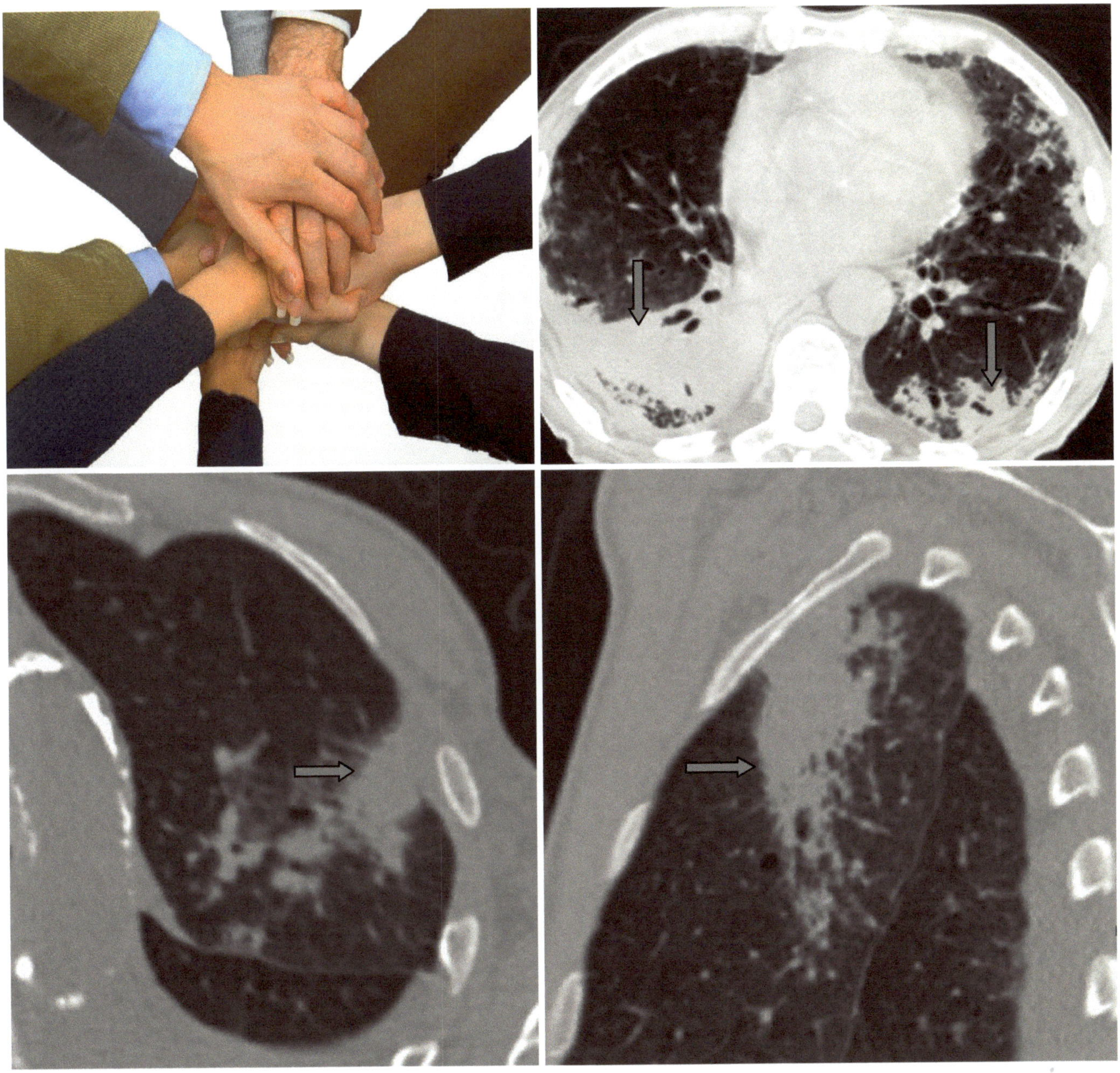

Air-space (alveolar, parenchymal) *consolidation* (↑) is a radiologic sign of increased lung opacity obscuring vascular and interstitial pattern. Consolidations may be divided to diffuse and focal, perihilar and peripheral, round, linear, and patchy. These features are important in differential diagnosis which is based on the nature of the substance that is replacing alveolar air: blood (hemorrhage), pus (exudates, pneumonia), water (transudate, edema), protein (secretions, lipoprotein), and cells (malignancies, COP). Air-filled bronchi are often seen under opacified lung parenchyma (air bronchogram sign). The presence or absence of air bronchograms cannot be considered as a proof of benign or malignant process existence.

A. Yudin, *Metaphorical Signs in Computed Tomography of Chest and Abdomen*,
DOI 10.1007/978-3-319-04013-4_4, © Springer International Publishing Switzerland 2014

Ground-Glass Opacity and Black Bronchus Sign

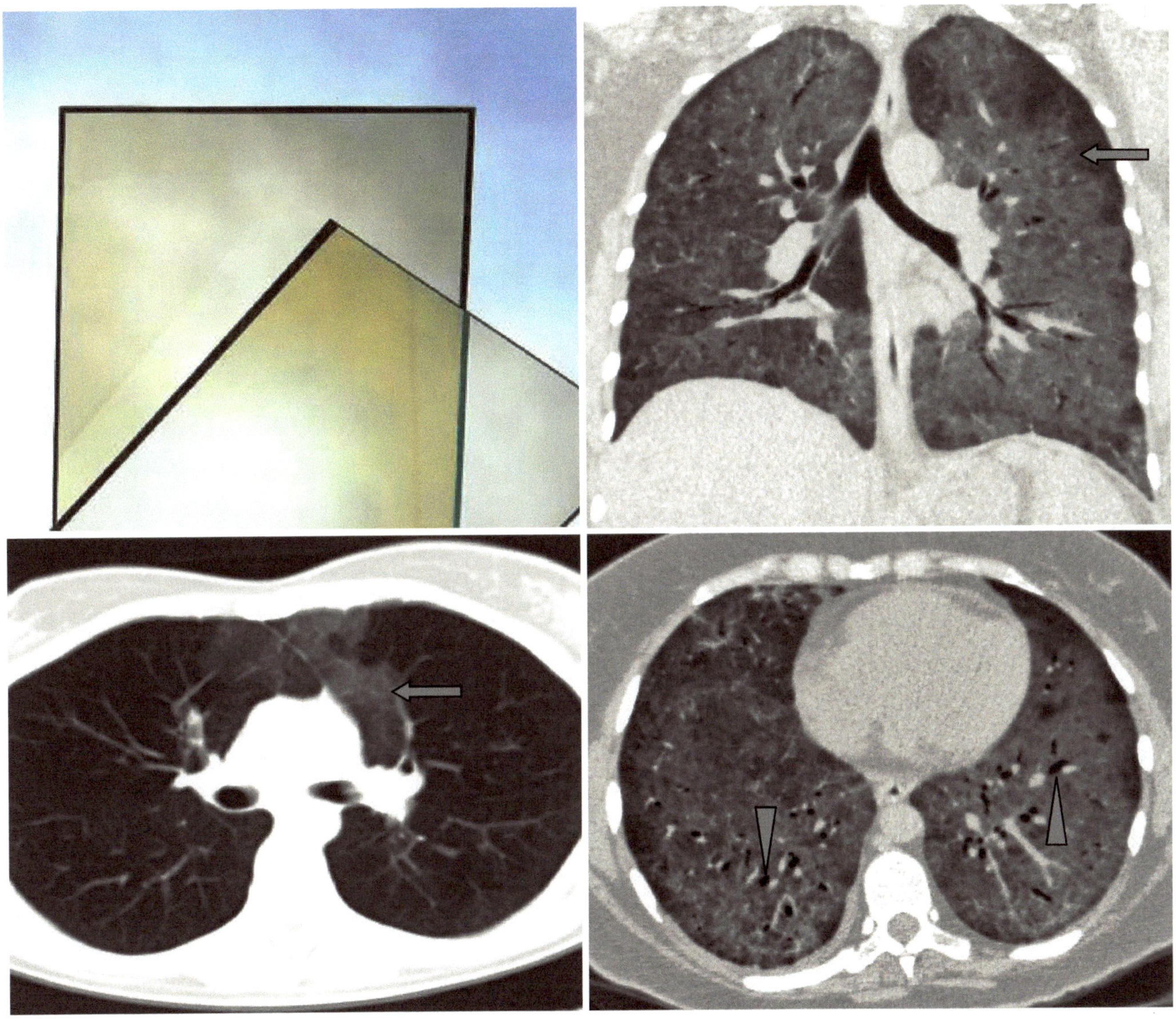

Ground-glass opacity (GGO) is a nonspecific finding which represents a hazy area of increased attenuation in the lung (↑) with preservation of bronchial and vascular margins. It may be caused by normal expiration, partial collapse of alveoli, increased capillary blood volume, partial filling of air spaces, or interstitial thickening. In patients with acute clinical symptoms, the presence of GGO reflects an active disease (e.g., pneumonia, edema, diffuse alveolar damage). In most patients with chronic symptoms, GGO also indicates active and potentially treatable stages of a long-lasting pathologic process (e.g., interstitial pneumonia, hypersensitivity pneumonitis, and sarcoidosis). GGO may also be found in patients with bronchoalveolar carcinoma that assumes dynamic control or morphological verification.

The bronchi filled with air are markedly seen against GGO unlike normal pulmonary tissue – the "black bronchus" sign (Δ).

A. Yudin, *Metaphorical Signs in Computed Tomography of Chest and Abdomen*,
DOI 10.1007/978-3-319-04013-4_5, © Springer International Publishing Switzerland 2014

Bat Wing, Butterfly, or Angel Wing Sign

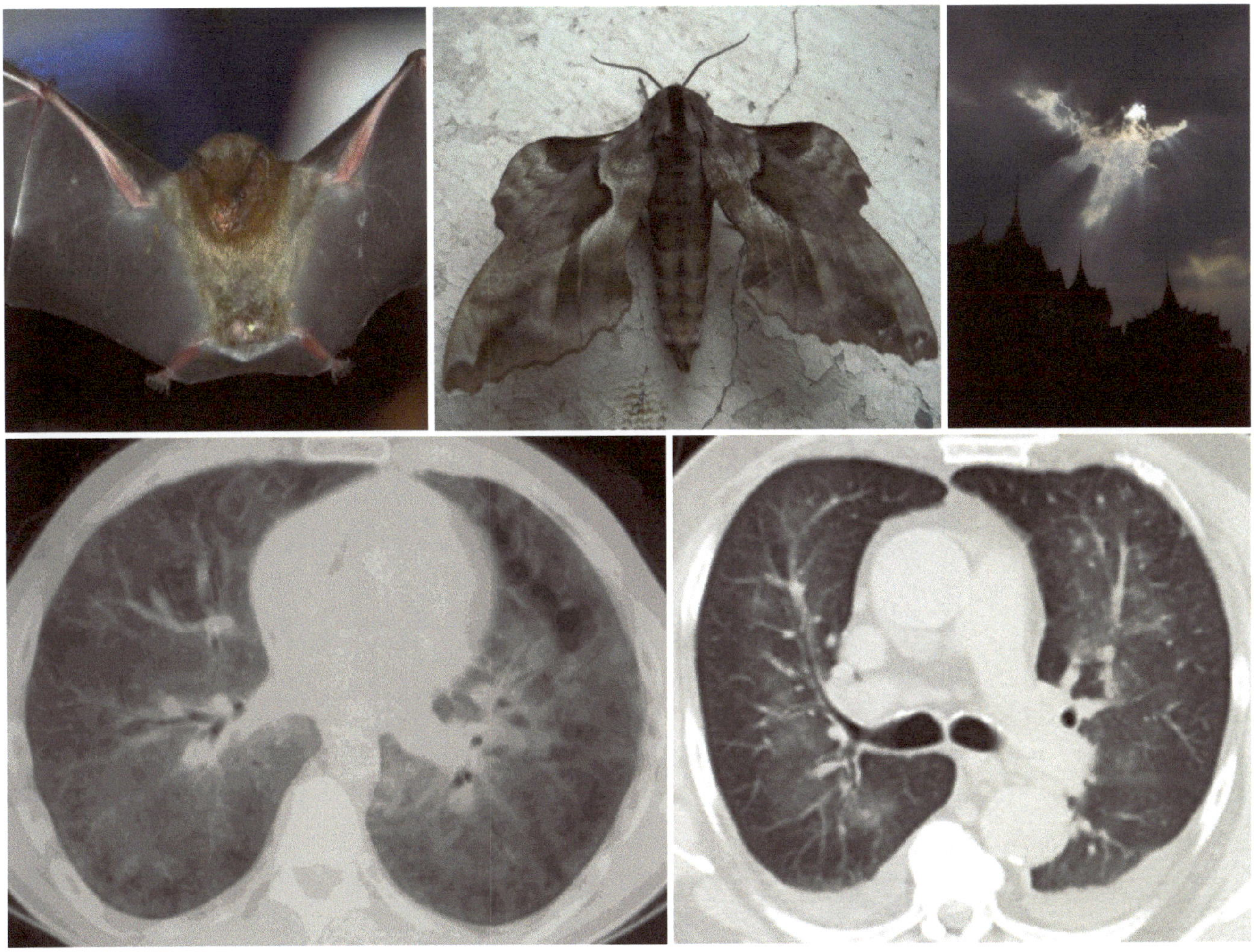

Air-space edema may be diffuse, multifocal, or patchy but mainly bilateral. Symmetrical perihilar ground-glass opacities sparing the cortex of the lungs (known as the "*bat wing*," "*butterfly*," or "*angel wing*" sign) may be seen sometimes and attributed to rapid accumulation of edema fluid. Similar pulmonary opacities can be found in patients with pneumonia, inhalation injuries, alveolar proteinosis, pulmonary hemorrhage, sarcoidosis, and bronchoalveolar carcinoma.

A. Yudin, *Metaphorical Signs in Computed Tomography of Chest and Abdomen*,
DOI 10.1007/978-3-319-04013-4_6, © Springer International Publishing Switzerland 2014

Crazy-Paving Sign

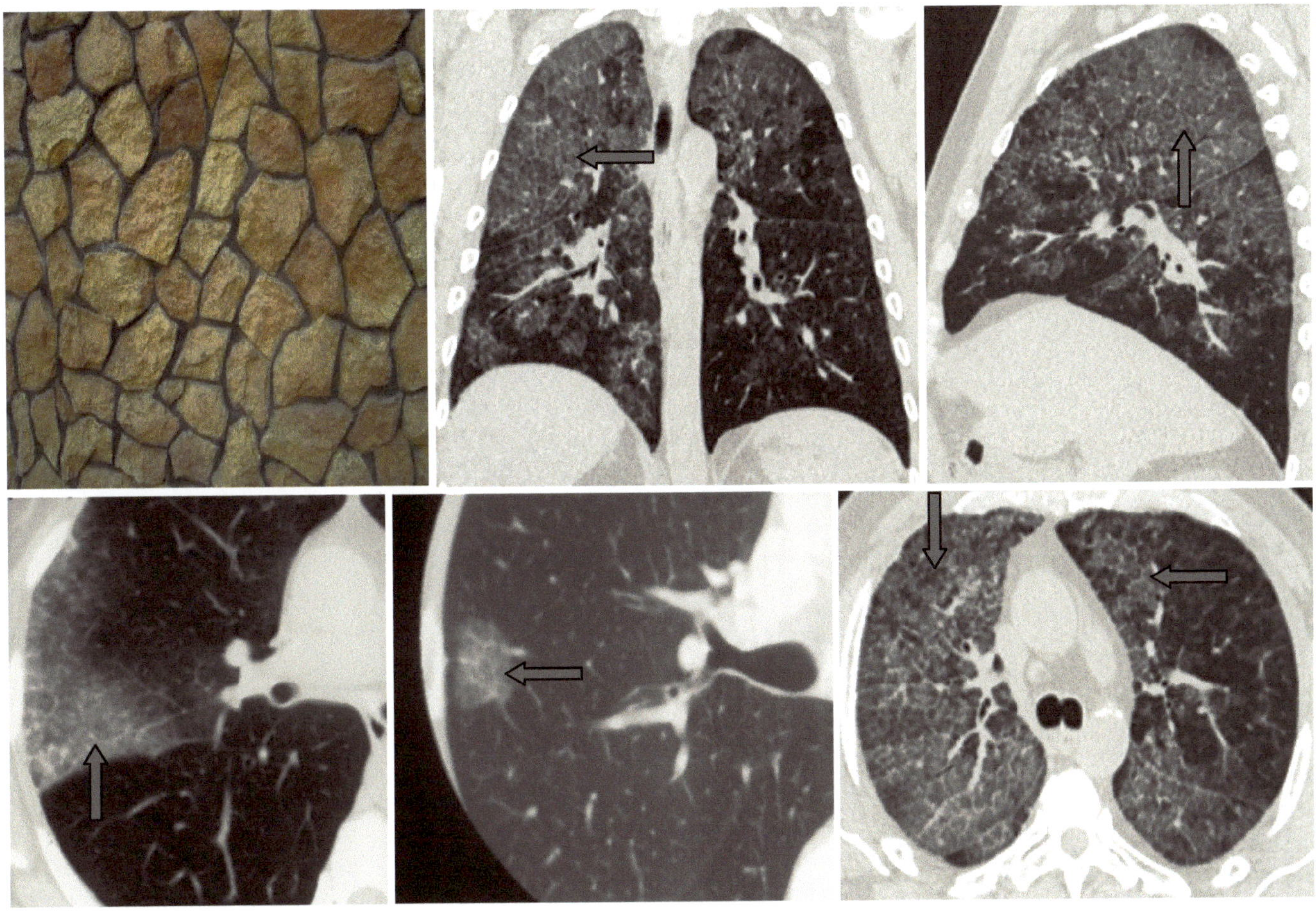

The combination of ground-glass opacity and fine reticular pattern is known as the "*crazy-paving*" sign (↑). It is a nonspecific finding that can be seen in a number of conditions both acute and chronic. Common causes of this sign include acute lung injury, pneumonia, pulmonary edema, hemorrhage, pulmonary alveolar proteinosis, bronchoalveolar carcinoma, interstitial pneumonia, and sarcoidosis. For proper diagnosis, biopsy or bronchoalveolar lavage may be warranted.

A. Yudin, *Metaphorical Signs in Computed Tomography of Chest and Abdomen*,
DOI 10.1007/978-3-319-04013-4_7, © Springer International Publishing Switzerland 2014

Honeycombing

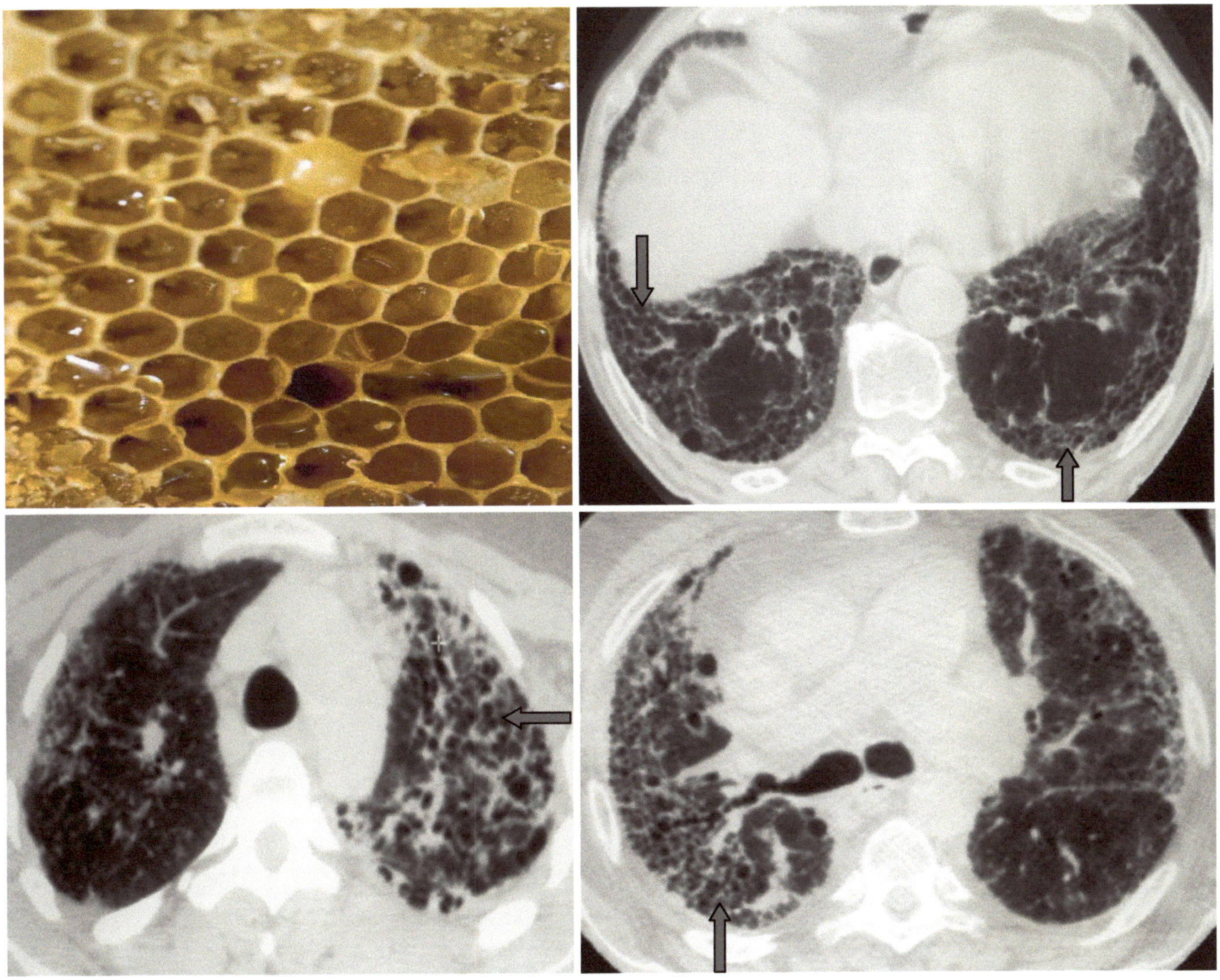

The term honeycomb lung is used to describe pathologic processes that cause appearance of multiple small, thick-walled cystic spaces. Clustered cystic air spaces (0.3–1.0 cm in diameter) or scattered cysts are usually visible beneath the pleural surfaces. In most cases, *honeycombing* (↑) reflects extensive lung fibrosis with total alveolar destruction (end-stage fibrosis). In up to 70 % of cases, honeycombing reflects the presence of usual interstitial pneumonia.

A. Yudin, *Metaphorical Signs in Computed Tomography of Chest and Abdomen*,
DOI 10.1007/978-3-319-04013-4_8, © Springer International Publishing Switzerland 2014

Vanishing Lung

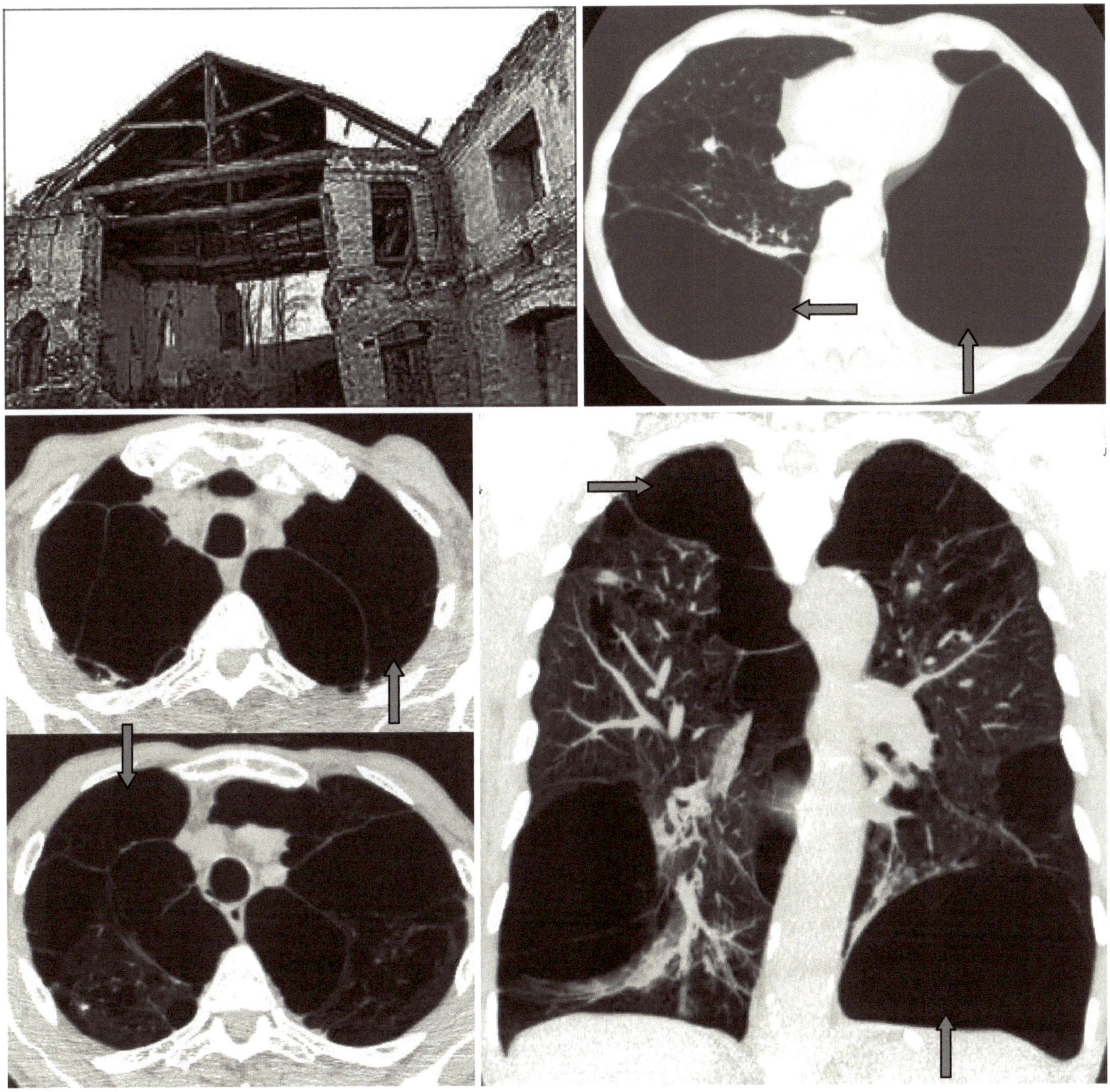

Vanishing lung (disappearing lung) also known as progressive (idiopathic) lung atrophy and idiopathic giant bullous emphysema is a rare disorder of unknown etiology used to describe lungs that seem to disappear on X-rays (↑). It is a progressive condition characterized by giant emphysematous bullae which commonly arise in the upper lobes and in the subpleural location. Bullae occupy at least one-third of hemithorax. They are usually seen in association with paraseptal and centrilobular emphysema, common in young men, mostly in smokers.

A. Yudin, *Metaphorical Signs in Computed Tomography of Chest and Abdomen*,
DOI 10.1007/978-3-319-04013-4_9, © Springer International Publishing Switzerland 2014

Mosaic Perfusion or Mosaic Lung Sign

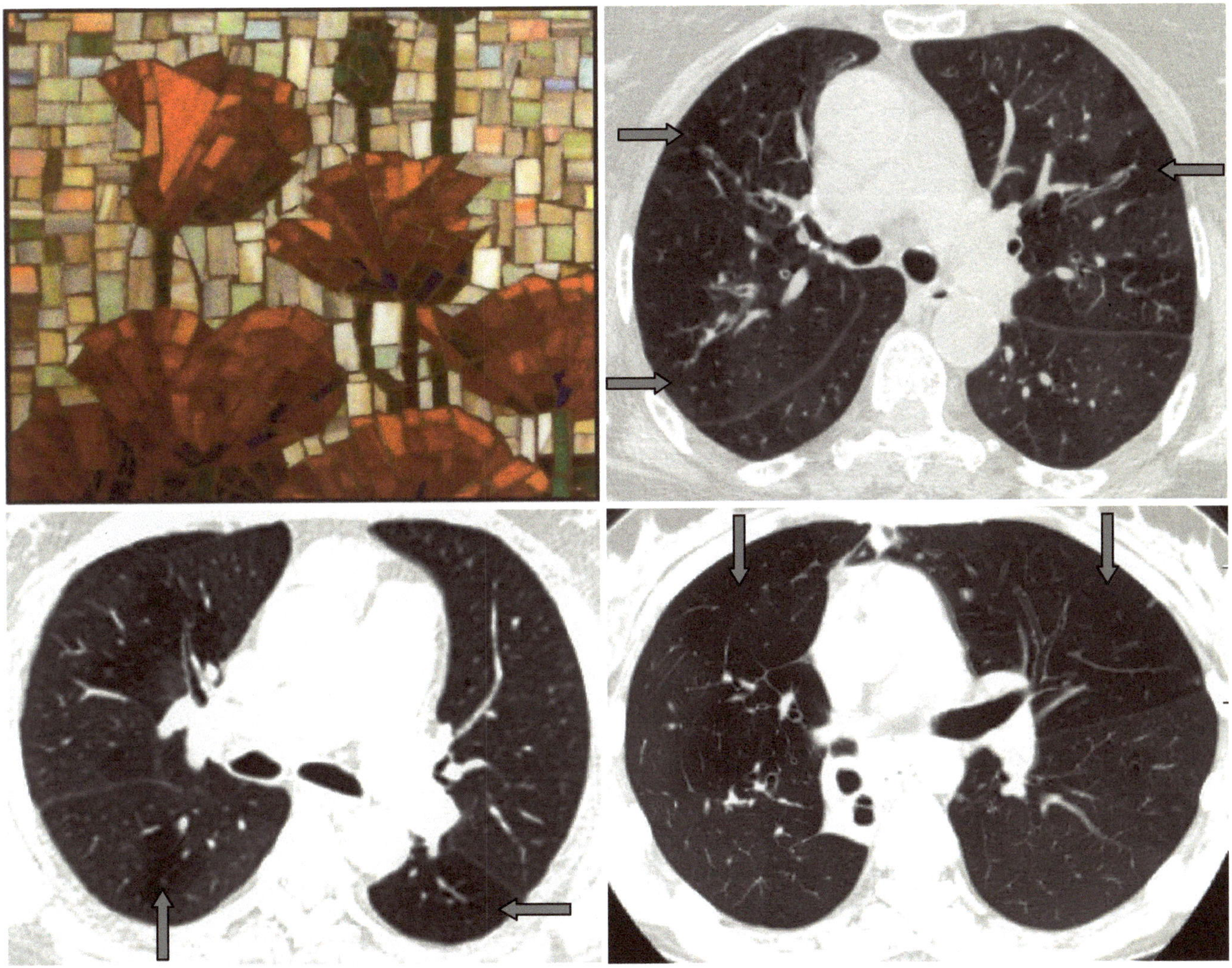

Mosaic perfusion (*mosaic attenuation*, the "*mosaic lung*" sign) refers to areas of decreased attenuation of lung parenchyma (↑) in the regions of reduced blood perfusion. The term "mosaic" reflects patchy distribution of abnormalities. This sign is usually seen in patients with small airways diseases (cystic fibrosis, bronchiolitis obliterans, and chronic obstructive lung disease) and pulmonary vascular disease (mosaic oligemia in chronic pulmonary embolism). In cases with mosaic perfusion, regional pulmonary artery branches are always reduced in size. This pattern gives opportunity to distinguish mosaic perfusion from ground-glass opacities.

A. Yudin, *Metaphorical Signs in Computed Tomography of Chest and Abdomen*,
DOI 10.1007/978-3-319-04013-4_10, © Springer International Publishing Switzerland 2014

Air Trapping

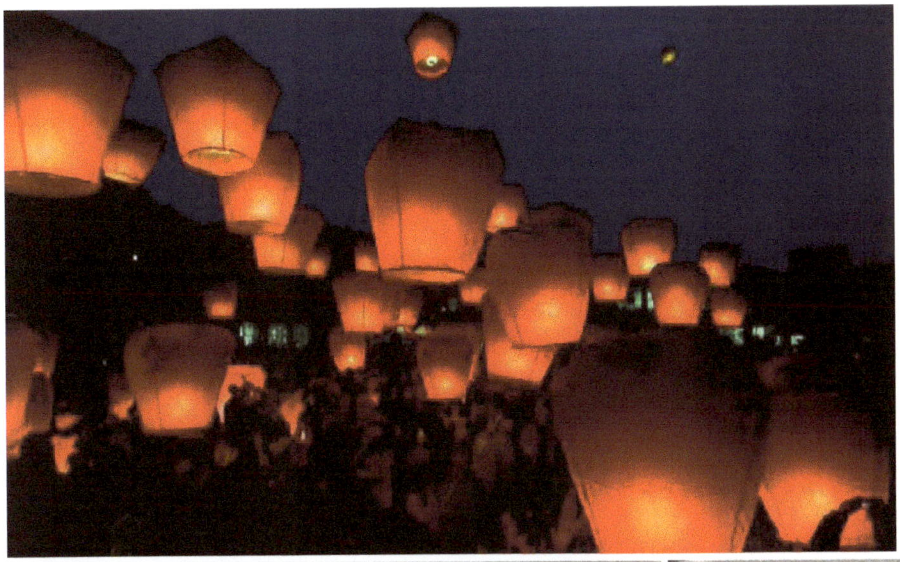

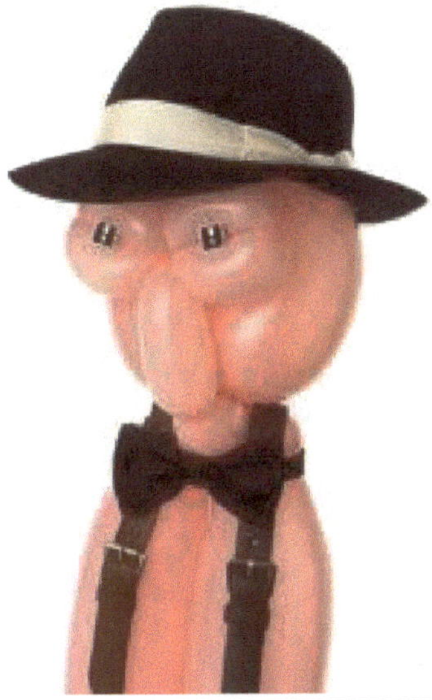

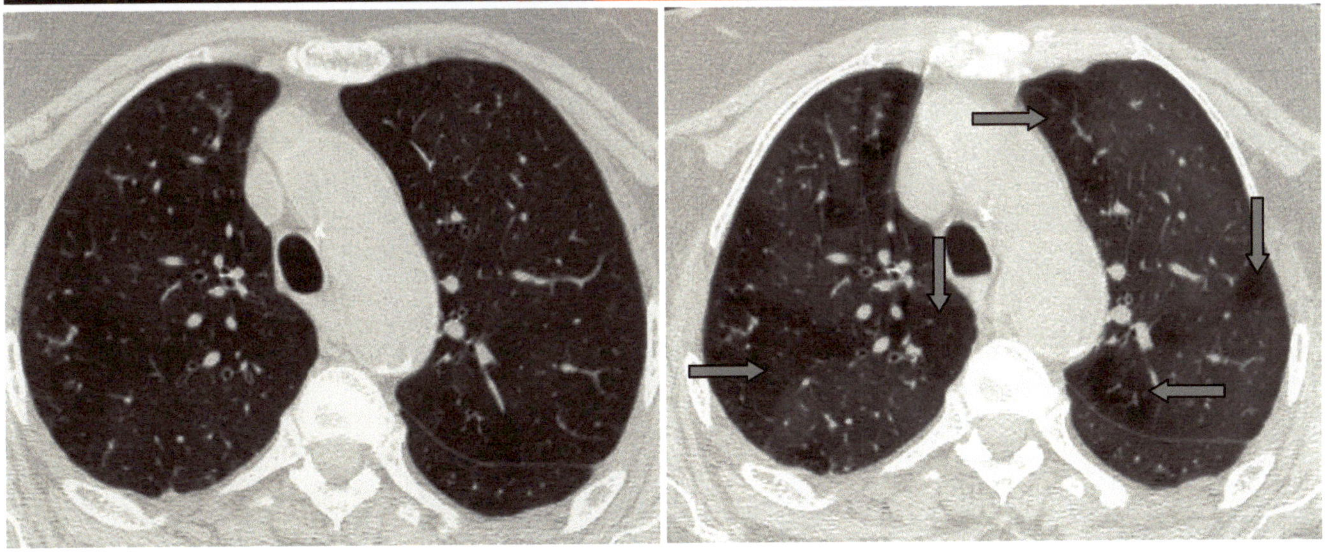

Air trapping or gas trapping (↑) refers to retention of excess gas in the secondary lobules of the lungs on expiratory scans (less than normal increase in attenuation of pulmonary parenchyma during expiration acquisition). The presence of this sign usually suggests small airways disease (bronchiolitis obliterans, chronic obstructive lung disease). Air trapping often coexists with other patterns of bronchial and bronchiolar pathology (mosaic perfusion, tree-in-bud, tram-tracking, and signet ring signs).

A. Yudin, *Metaphorical Signs in Computed Tomography of Chest and Abdomen*,
DOI 10.1007/978-3-319-04013-4_11, © Springer International Publishing Switzerland 2014

Swiss Cheese Appearance

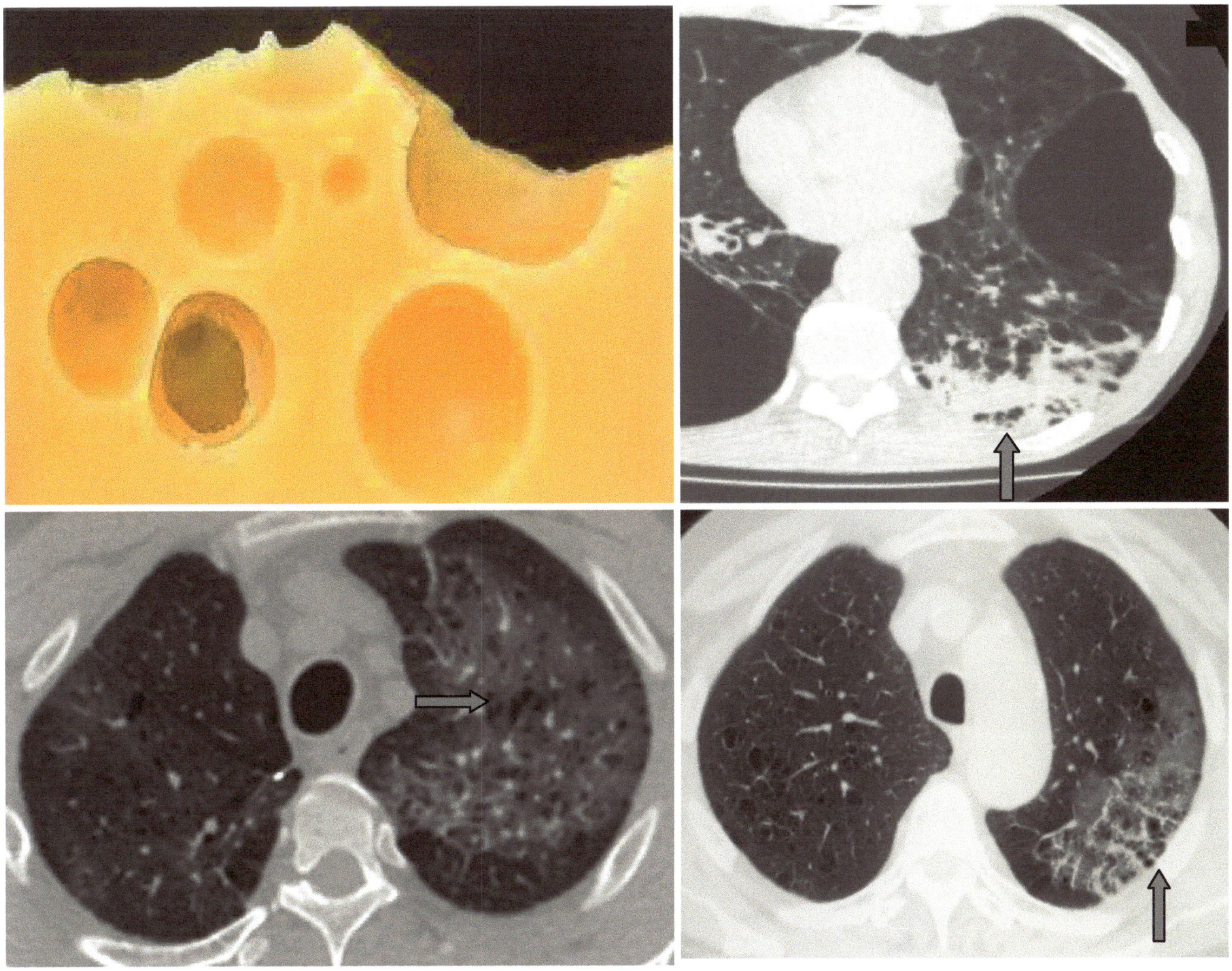

Pneumonia is the most frequent acute complication of chronic obstructive pulmonary disease. In patients with emphysema consolidation of the pulmonary tissue caused by pneumonia may look nonuniformly "perforated" so forming the "*Swiss cheese*" *appearance* (↑). The presence of emphysema often leads to wrong diagnosis of interstitial lung disease in such cases.

A. Yudin, *Metaphorical Signs in Computed Tomography of Chest and Abdomen*,
DOI 10.1007/978-3-319-04013-4_12, © Springer International Publishing Switzerland 2014

Feeding Vessel Sign or Fruits on the Branch Sign

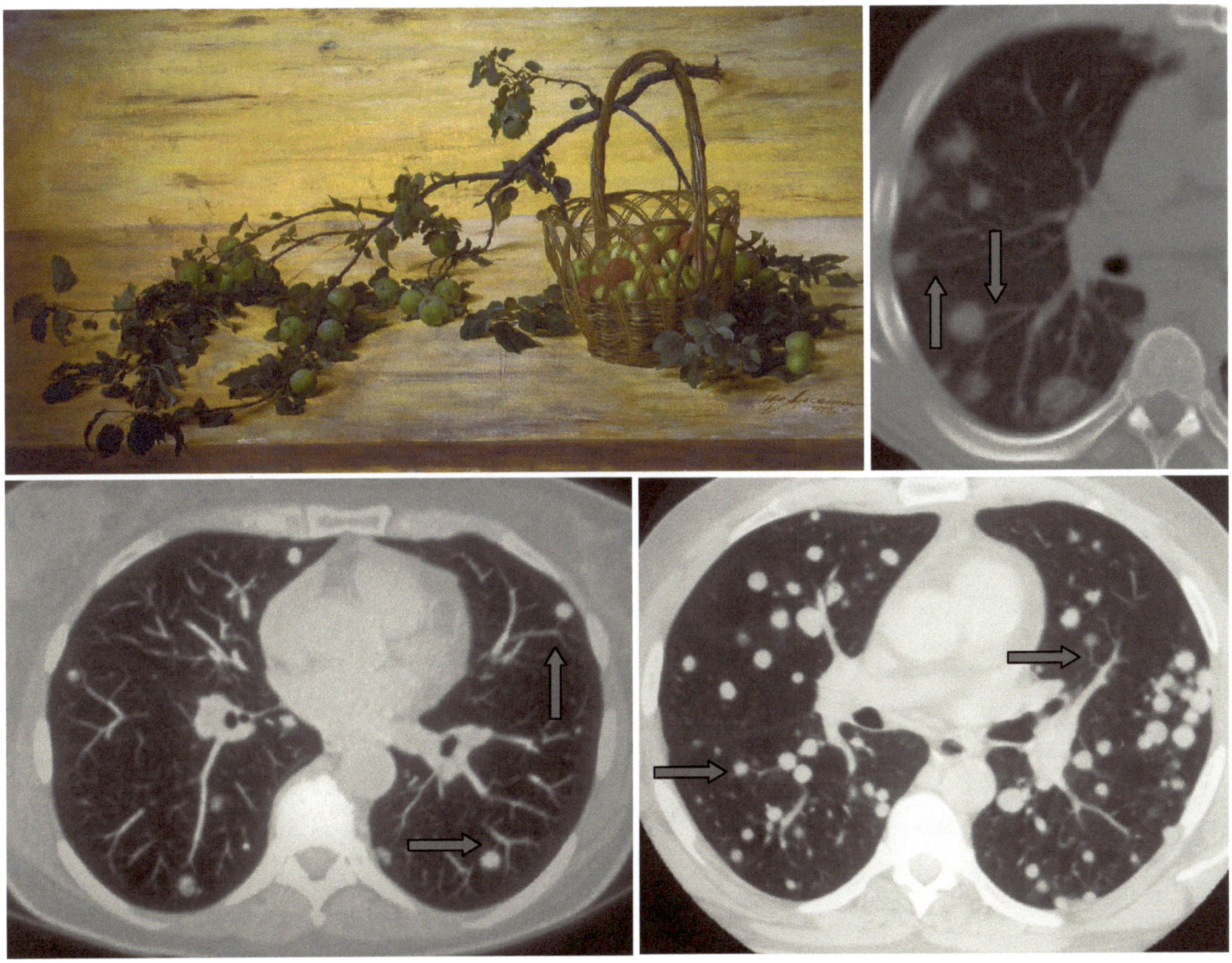

The "*feeding vessel*" sign also known as the "*fruits on the branch*" sign (↑) refers to the branch of a pulmonary artery leading directly to a nodule or a mass. This sign is most often seen with pulmonary metastases and septic embolism and also frequently occurs in infarcts and arteriovenous fistulas. It is rarely seen in lung carcinomas and granulomas.

A. Yudin, *Metaphorical Signs in Computed Tomography of Chest and Abdomen*,
DOI 10.1007/978-3-319-04013-4_13, © Springer International Publishing Switzerland 2014

Snowstorm Sign and Cannonball Metastases

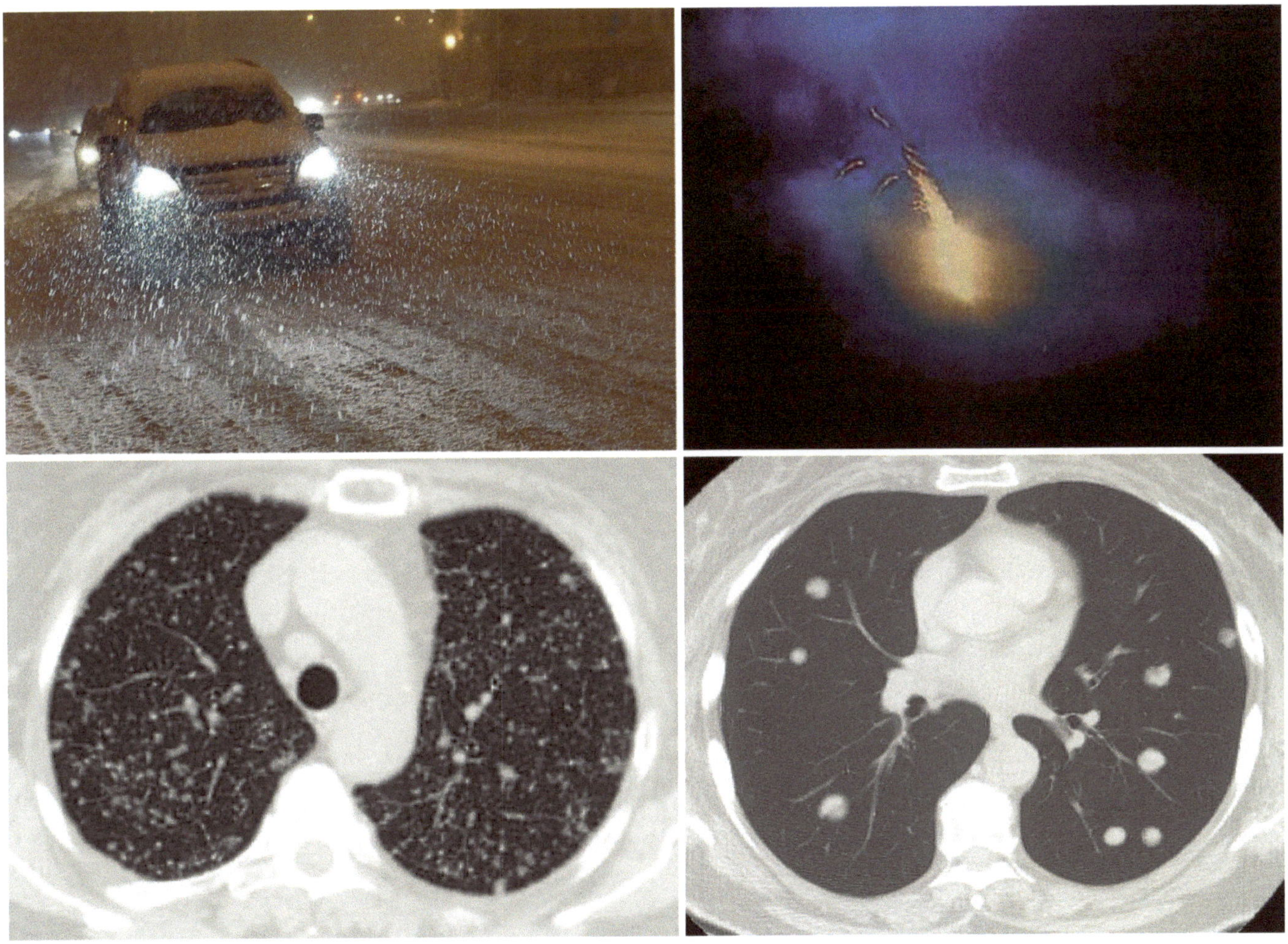

Lung metastases are characterized by casual (random) distribution. The form and the size of the nodules can vary within appreciable limits. If the nodules have small (miliary) sizes and their quantity is innumerable (the "*snowstorm*" sign), the metastases of vascular tumors (thyroid gland carcinoma, renal cell carcinoma, adenocarcinoma, sarcoma) usually take place (left images). If the nodes have a big size and are accurately outlined, then they are called *cannonball metastases*. Such metastases are characteristic of tumors of the gastrointestinal tract and genitourinary sphere (right images).

A. Yudin, *Metaphorical Signs in Computed Tomography of Chest and Abdomen*,
DOI 10.1007/978-3-319-04013-4_14, © Springer International Publishing Switzerland 2014

Air Bronchograms and Pseudocavitations

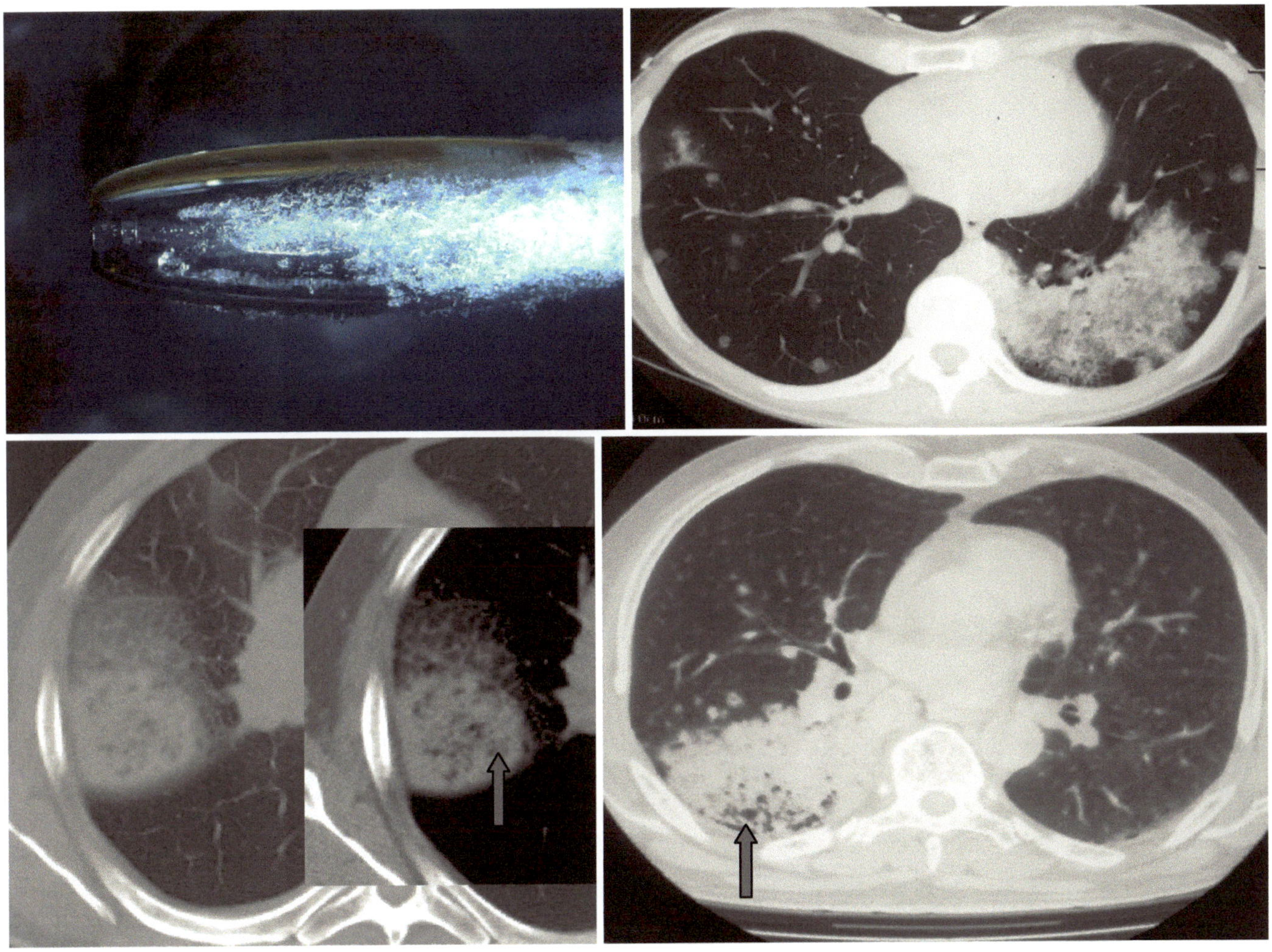

Air bronchograms and *pseudocavitations* (↑) are often visible in adenocarcinomas (bronchoalveolar carcinomas) and seldom occur in benign lung lesions. Air bronchograms can be also found in pneumonias, round atelectases, inside conglomerate masses in silicosis, and sarcoidosis. Fine lucencies against a neoplasm represent cystic sites filled with air (pseudocavitations).

A. Yudin, *Metaphorical Signs in Computed Tomography of Chest and Abdomen*,
DOI 10.1007/978-3-319-04013-4_15, © Springer International Publishing Switzerland 2014

Halo Sign

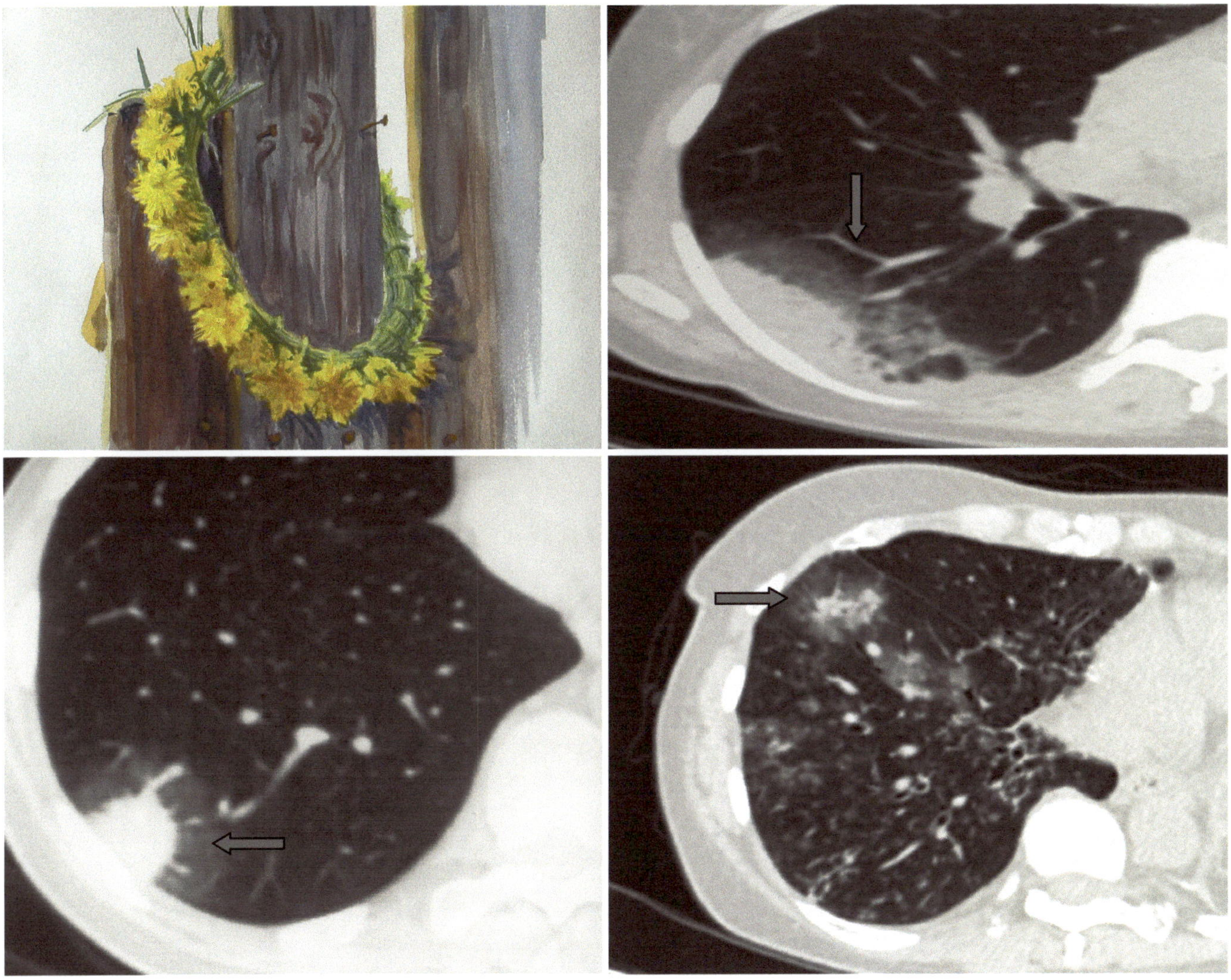

The rim formed by a zone of "ground-glass" density (↑), which surrounds a consolidation or a group of nodules in a lung (the "*halo*" sign), can be seen in patients with aspergillosis (less common with other infections) and also around adenocarcinomas (especially bronchoalveolar carcinomas). In aspergillosis, the halo is caused by hemorrhages. The halo around adenocarcinoma is formed by the tumor growth in the interstitial tissue.

A. Yudin, *Metaphorical Signs in Computed Tomography of Chest and Abdomen*,
DOI 10.1007/978-3-319-04013-4_16, © Springer International Publishing Switzerland 2014

Corona Radiata or Corona Maligna and Pleural Tail Sign

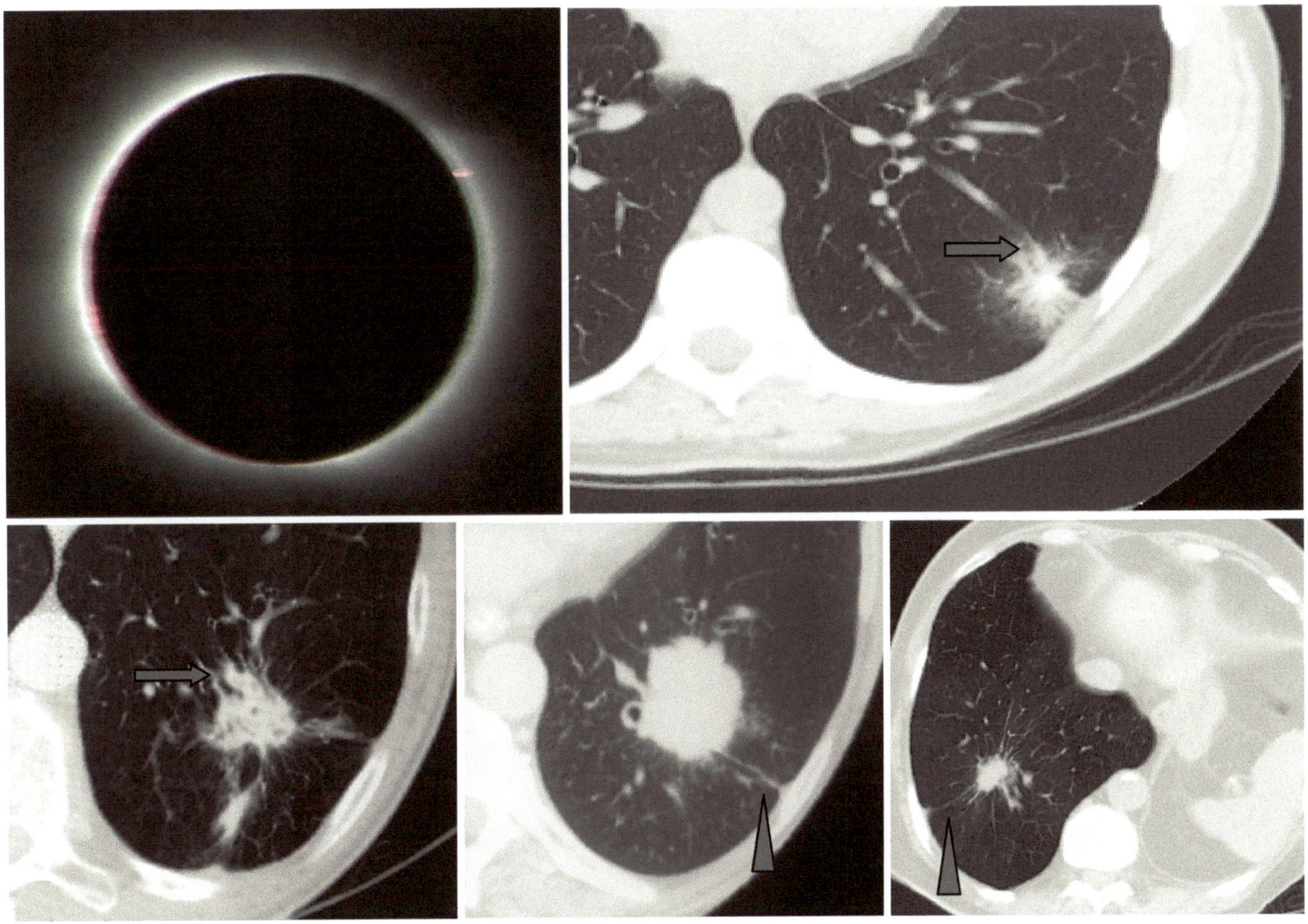

Primary malignant neoplasms of lungs often have weakly outlined rough contours with spicules forming "*corona radiata*" or "*corona maligna*" (↑). 90 % of nodes with spicules and only 20 % of nodes with well-defined even contours prove to be malignant. "Corona radiata" usually corresponds to a desmoplastic reaction, but the tumor invasion can also be present. Additionally, detection of the thin strip propagating to the pleura (Δ) with a local triangular protrusion is possible (the "*pleural tail*" sign). This sign also reflects the presence of fibrosis and can be detected equally with benign and malignant formations. Concerning malignant process "corona radiata" is more specific than the "pleural tail" sign.

A. Yudin, *Metaphorical Signs in Computed Tomography of Chest and Abdomen*,
DOI 10.1007/978-3-319-04013-4_17, © Springer International Publishing Switzerland 2014

Positive Bronchus Sign

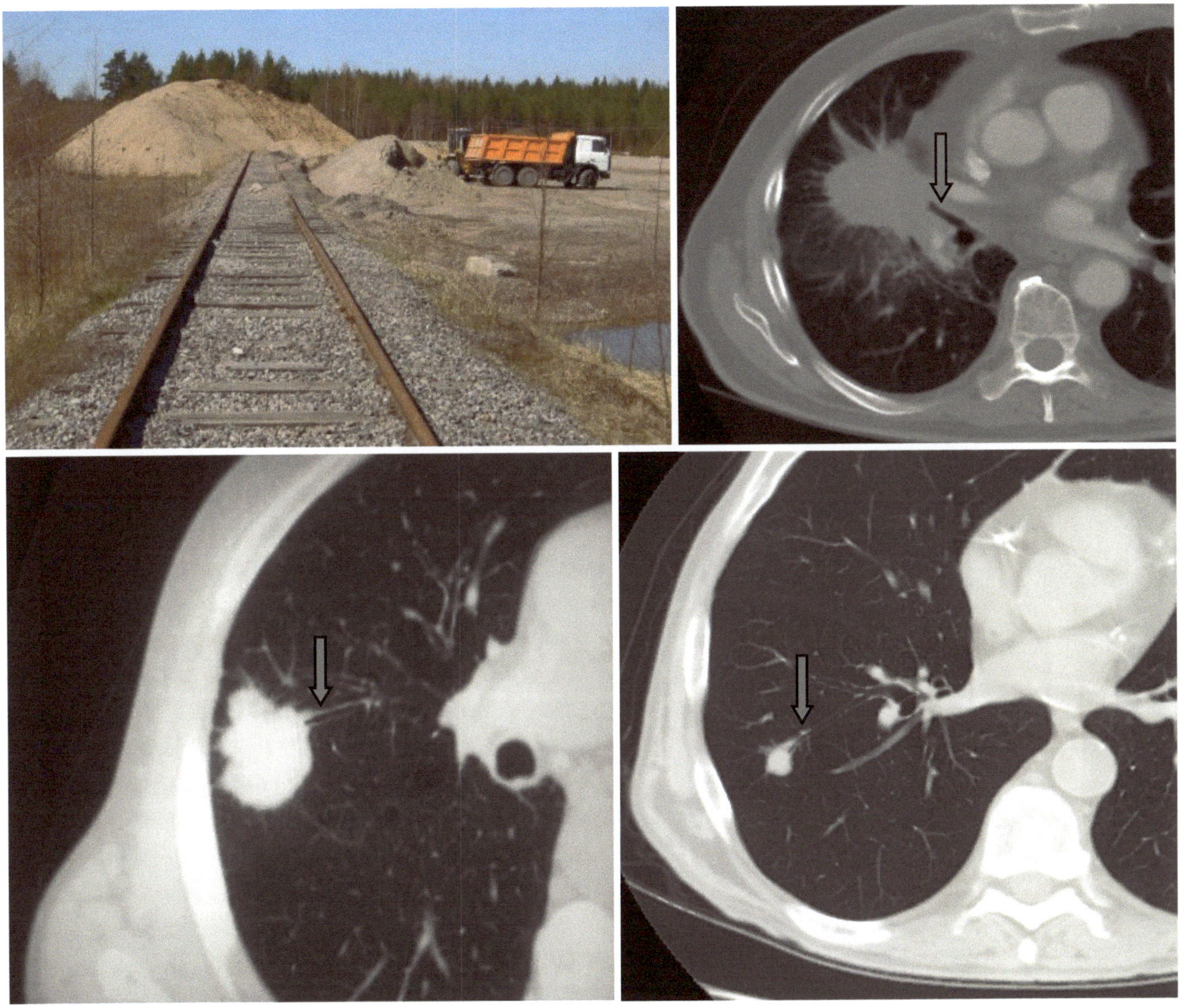

Bronchoscopy with biopsy plays a limited role in verification of peripheral lesions of the lungs (about 30 % with nodes smaller than 3 cm in diameter). Efficiency of bronchoscopy considerably rises if the bronchus tends directly to the tumor or is visible in it forming on tomograms the "*positive bronchus*" sign (↑).

A. Yudin, *Metaphorical Signs in Computed Tomography of Chest and Abdomen*,
DOI 10.1007/978-3-319-04013-4_18, © Springer International Publishing Switzerland 2014

Umbilical Retraction Sign or Rigler Incisura

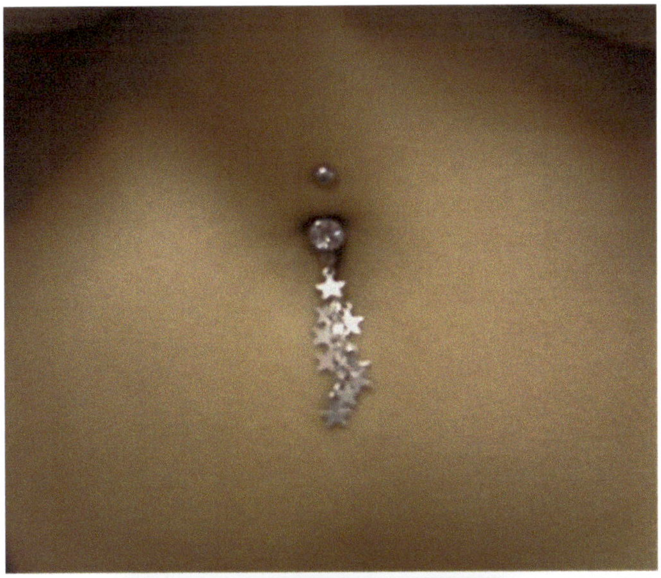

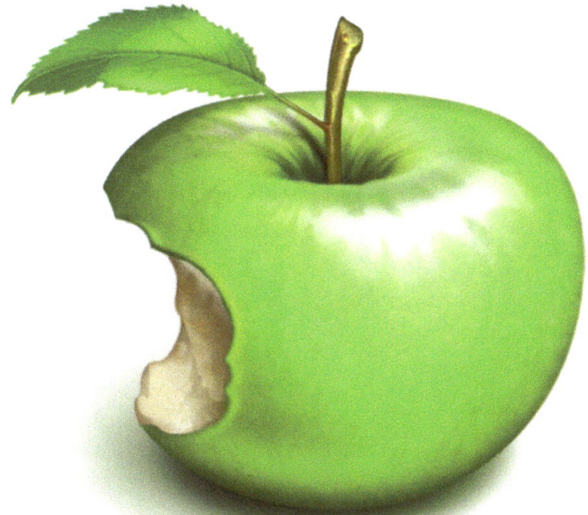

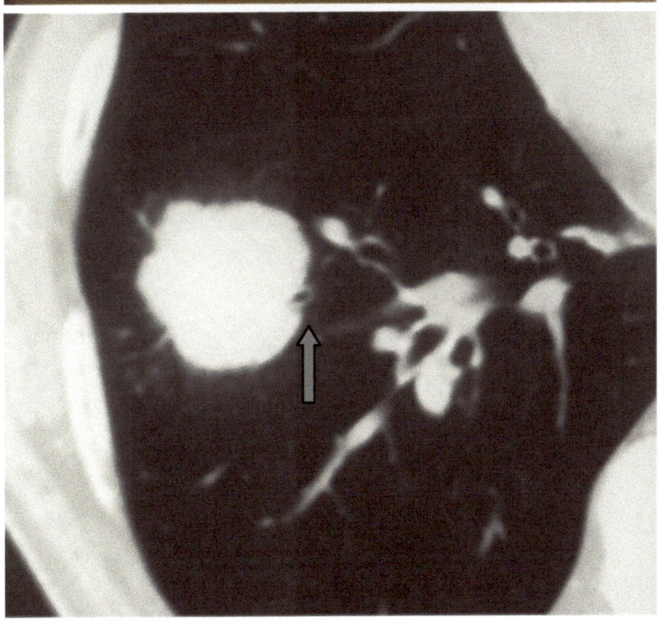

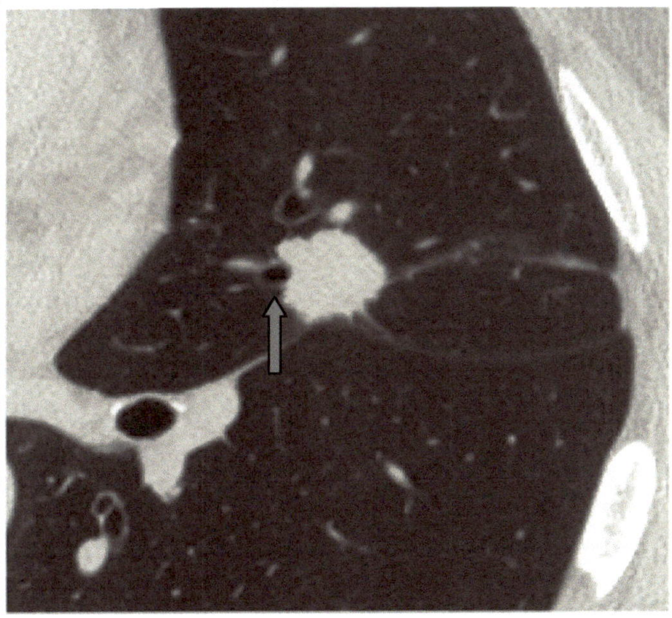

In classic radiology, the "*umbilical retraction*" sign *or Rigler incisura* is described as a retraction of the tumor contour in the form of a notch caused by tumor overgrowth around the bronchus and pulmonary artery (↑). In contrast to the "positive bronchus" sign, the likelihood of morphological verification during bronchoscopy in such a situation is questionable.

A. Yudin, *Metaphorical Signs in Computed Tomography of Chest and Abdomen*,
DOI 10.1007/978-3-319-04013-4_19, © Springer International Publishing Switzerland 2014

Popcorn Sign and Bull's Eye Calcifications

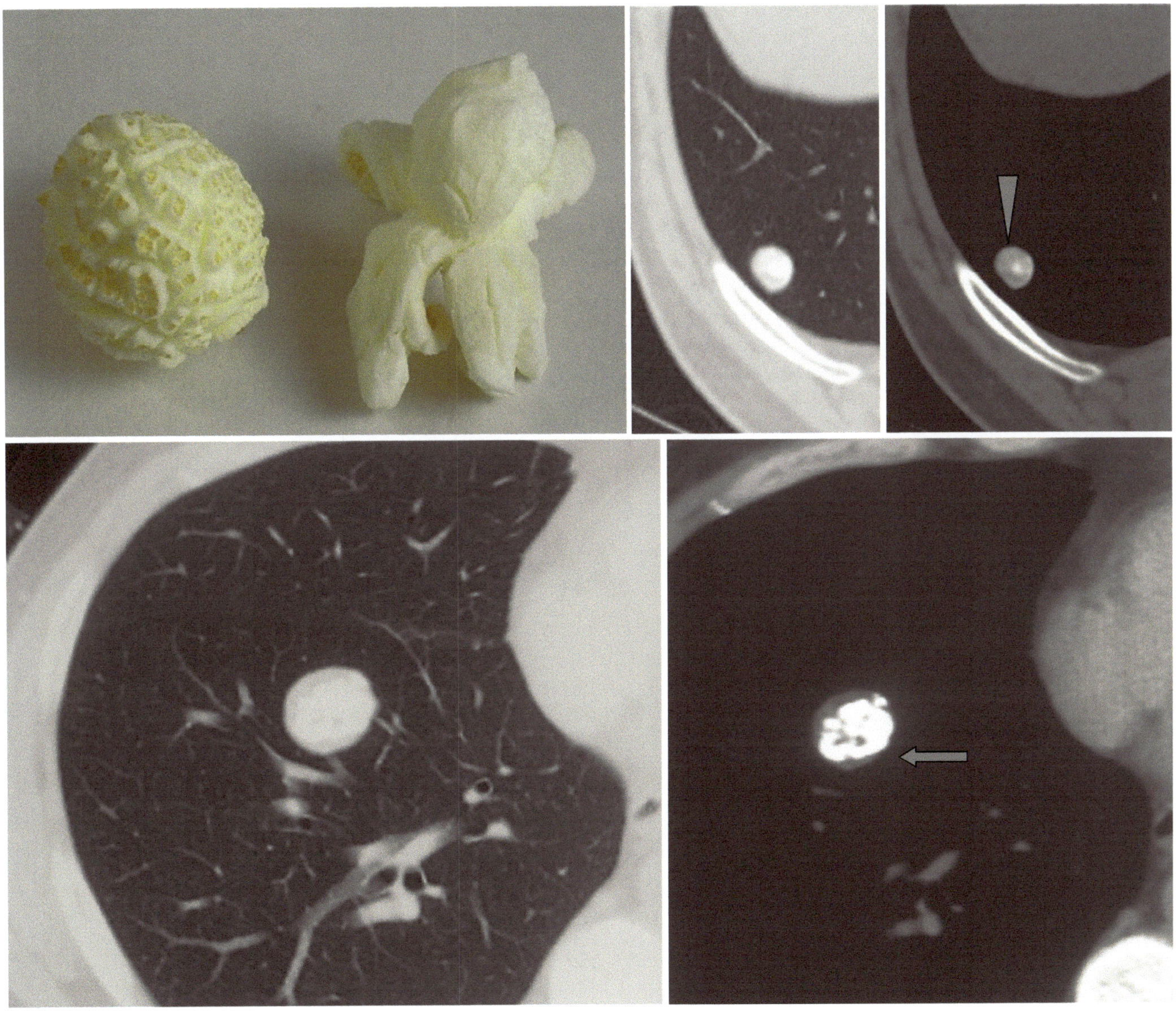

The conglomerate of formless calcifications occupying the central part of a lung nodule forms the "*popcorn*" sign (↑) characteristic of hamartoma. Dot-like calcification in the center of a nodule is known as the *bull's eye calcification* (Δ) occurring in hamartomas and histoplasmomas, also possible in any granuloma.

A. Yudin, *Metaphorical Signs in Computed Tomography of Chest and Abdomen*,
DOI 10.1007/978-3-319-04013-4_20, © Springer International Publishing Switzerland 2014

Target Calcification Sign

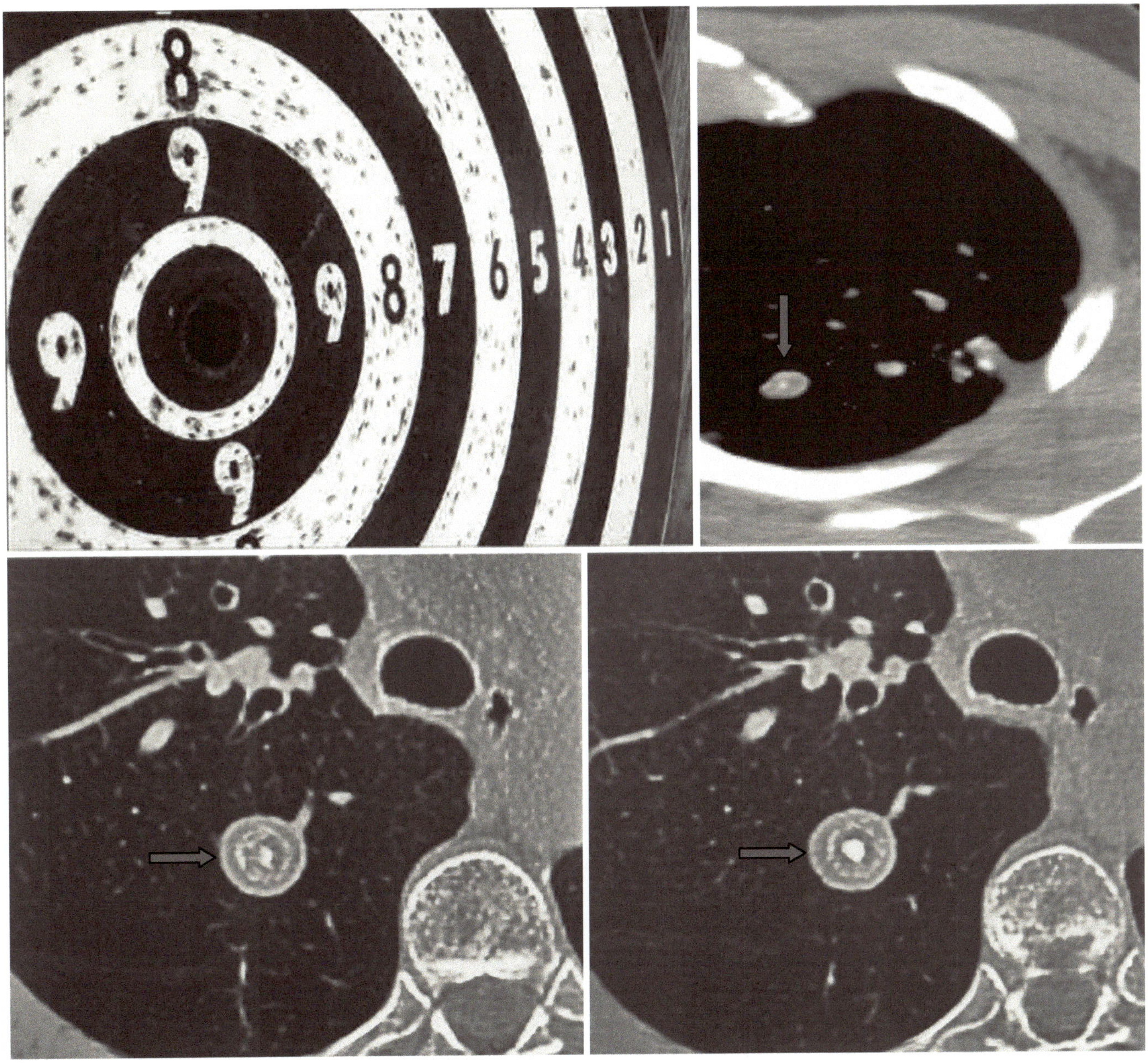

Concentric (laminar) calcification in a lung nodule known as the "*target*" sign (↑) occurs in tuberculomas and histoplasmosis.

A. Yudin, *Metaphorical Signs in Computed Tomography of Chest and Abdomen*,
DOI 10.1007/978-3-319-04013-4_21, © Springer International Publishing Switzerland 2014

Satellite Foci and Galaxy Sign

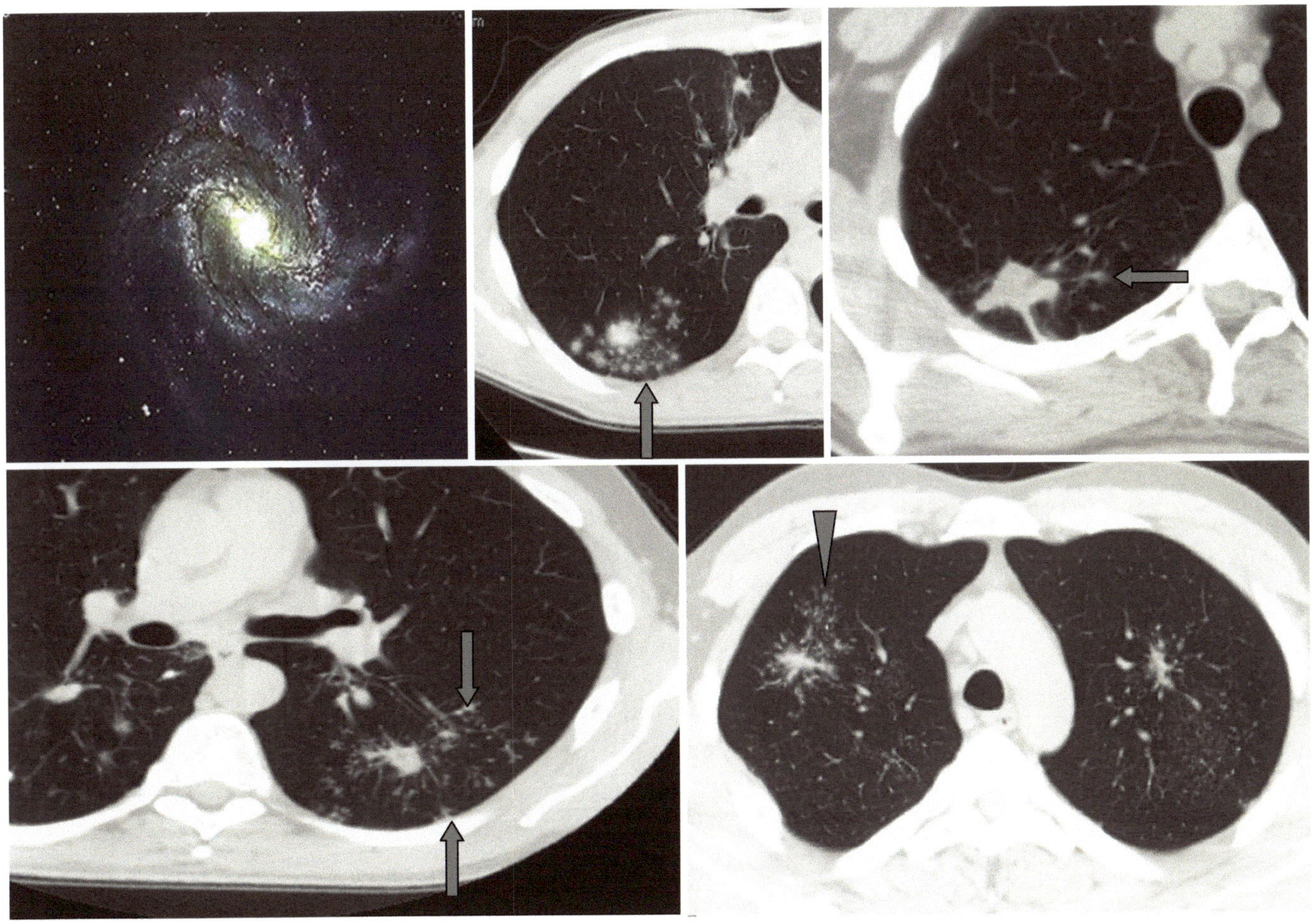

The *satellite foci* (↑) can be found near lung nodules, and usually they are a sign of benign process (granulomatoses, tuberculosis). In patients with sarcoidosis the satellite nodules are described as the "*galaxy*" sign (Δ). In rare cases the satellite nodules can also be found at carcinomas.

A. Yudin, *Metaphorical Signs in Computed Tomography of Chest and Abdomen*,
DOI 10.1007/978-3-319-04013-4_22, © Springer International Publishing Switzerland 2014

Rounded Atelectasis, Comet-Tail Sign, and Crow's Foot Sign

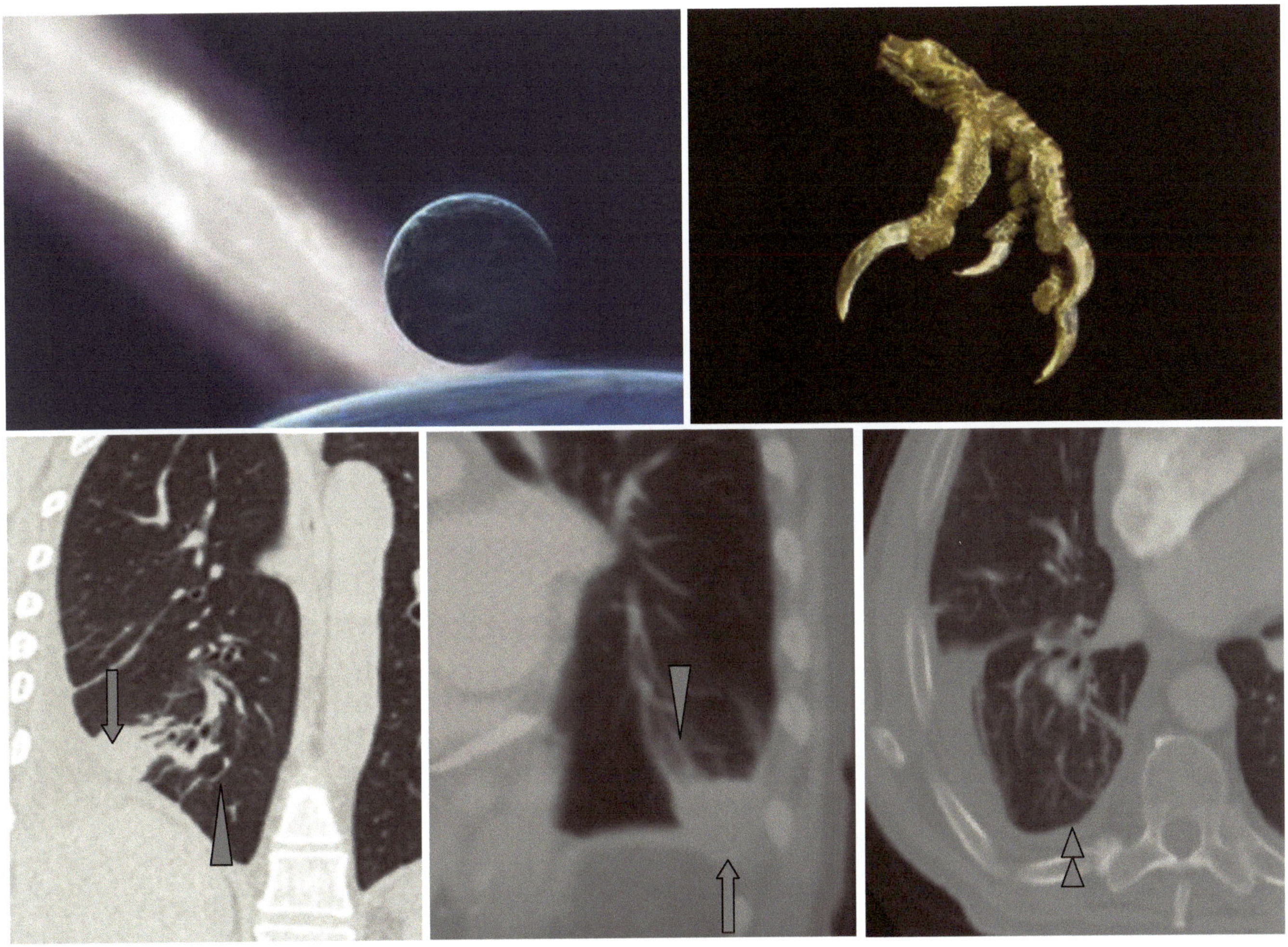

Rounded atelectasis (↑) represents a local collapse of a lung in the form of a ball-shaped zone of consolidation usually combined with pathologic changes of the pleura and architectonical disturbance of the surrounding pulmonary tissue. In the formation of rounded atelectasis, the proximally located vessels, bronchi, and interstitial tissue fold and twist which results in a comet-tail appearance on images – the "*comet-tail*" sign (Δ). A group of randomly located interstitial bundles in the lungs predominantly directed to the thickened pleura can precede the formation of rounded atelectasis mimicking a bird's paw – the "*crow's foot*" sign (►►). The local thickenings of the pleura, the "comet-tail" sign, and the rounded atelectasis quite often occur in asbestosis but are not specific for this disease.

A. Yudin, *Metaphorical Signs in Computed Tomography of Chest and Abdomen*,
DOI 10.1007/978-3-319-04013-4_23, © Springer International Publishing Switzerland 2014

Tree-in-Bud Sign

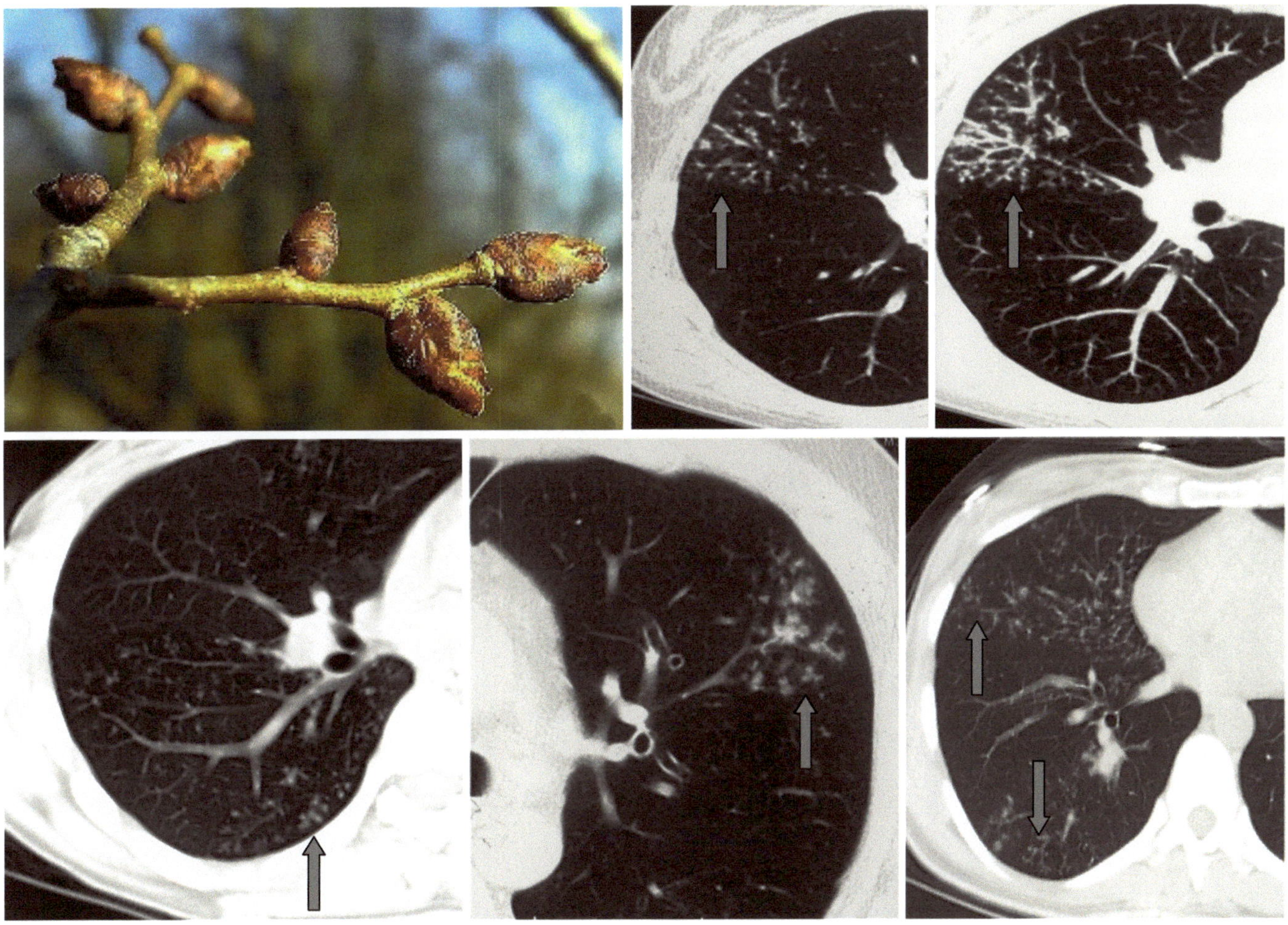

In intralobular distribution of nodules, the "*tree-in-bud*" sign can be seen (↑) which is characterized as the presence of small well-defined foci at the ends of linear intralobular structures. This sign almost always indicates the presence of dilated and filled with some substrate (mucus, detritus, pus, cellular elements) intralobular bronchioles. In overwhelming majority of cases, this sign testifies the existence of intrabronchiolar infection (tubercular, bacterial, fungal) and extremely rare intrabronchiolar spread of a tumor. Accordingly, for specified diagnostics, it is expedient to consider performance of bronchoalveolar lavage, sputum analysis, and PCR diagnostics.

A. Yudin, *Metaphorical Signs in Computed Tomography of Chest and Abdomen*,
DOI 10.1007/978-3-319-04013-4_24,

Air Crescent Sign

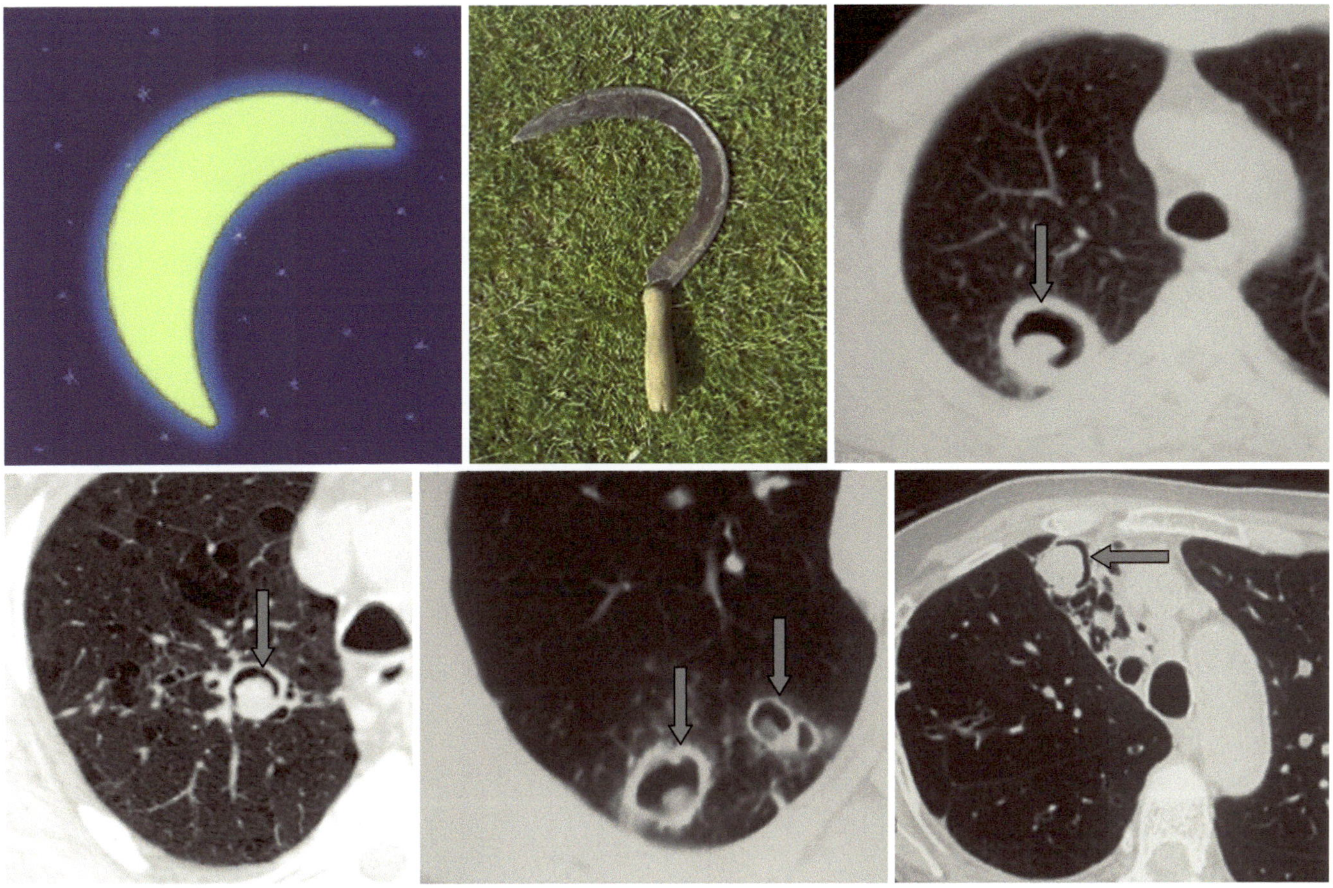

In lung cavities of any origin (cysts, caverns, tumors, emphysema, and so forth), the soft tissue nodes can be visualized which are delimited at the edge by a crescent collection of air – the "*air crescent*" sign (↑). The most frequent reason for the occurrence of this sign is aspergilloma (mycetoma), but there may be other reasons which are much less frequent (septic infarct, a carcinoma in a cyst, a cavitary carcinoma, a clot in a cyst or a cavity, echinococcosis, sputum in a cystic bronchiectasia, papillomatosis of lungs, gangrene, Rasmussen aneurysm).

A. Yudin, *Metaphorical Signs in Computed Tomography of Chest and Abdomen*,
DOI 10.1007/978-3-319-04013-4_25, © Springer International Publishing Switzerland 2014

Signet Ring Sign, Tram-Tracking Sign, String of Pearls, and Cluster of Grapes

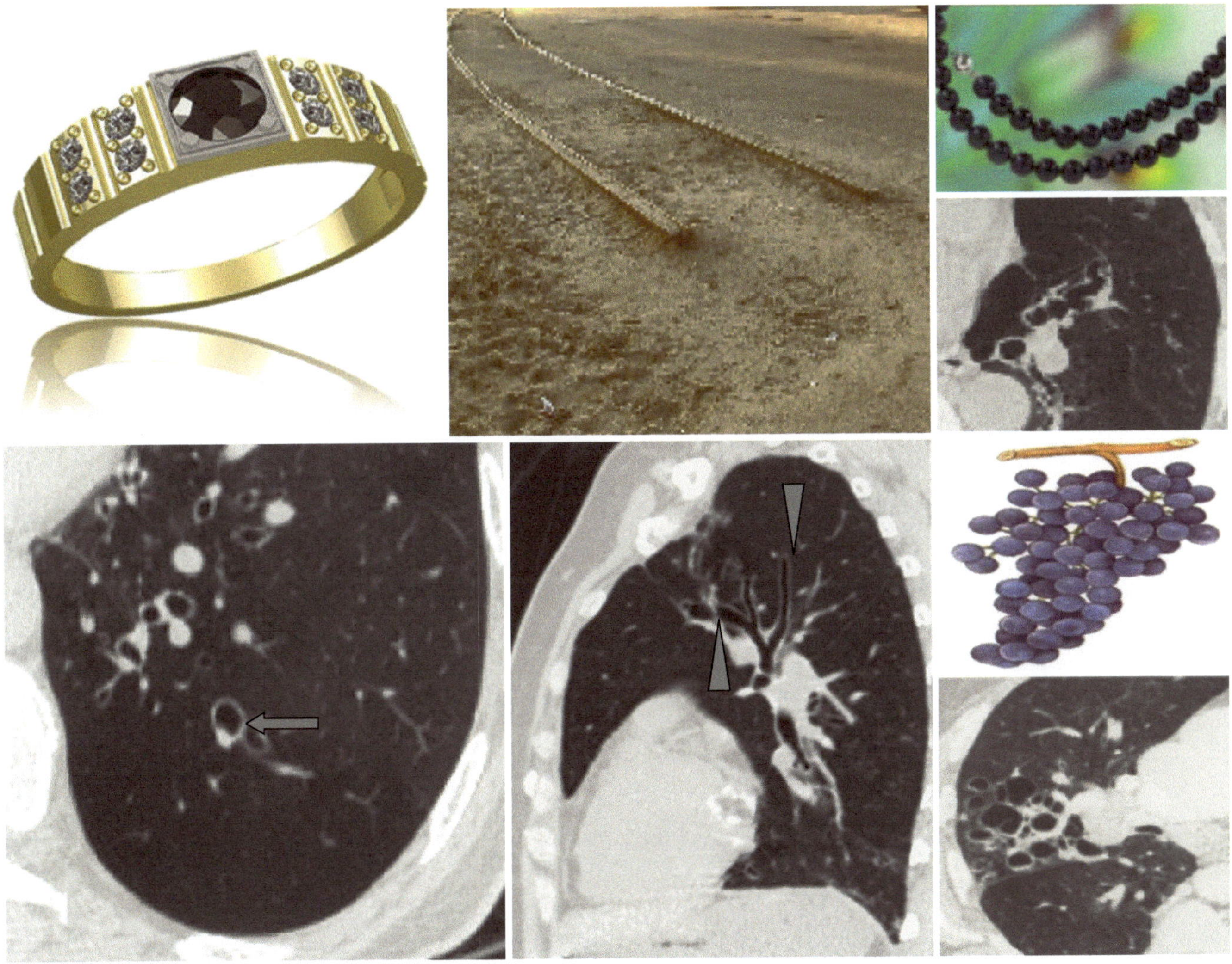

These are the signs of bronchiectasia. In true bronchiectasia, the diameter of a bronchial lumen which is perpendicular to the tomogram plane exceeds the diameter of the adjacent pulmonary artery branch (↑) more than 1.5 times (the "*signet ring*" sign). Parallel walls of the bronchi in cylinder bronchiectasias when visualized in the plane of tomographic image form the "*tram-tracking*" sign (Δ) because there is no normal narrowing of a bronchial lumen to the periphery. Varicose bronchiectasias in the tomographic plane look like a chain or the "*string of pearls*" (right upper images). The group of cystic bronchiectasias can create a view of the "*cluster of grapes*" on CT (right lower images).

A. Yudin, *Metaphorical Signs in Computed Tomography of Chest and Abdomen*,
DOI 10.1007/978-3-319-04013-4_26, © Springer International Publishing Switzerland 2014

Finger-in-Glove or Hand-in-Glove Sign

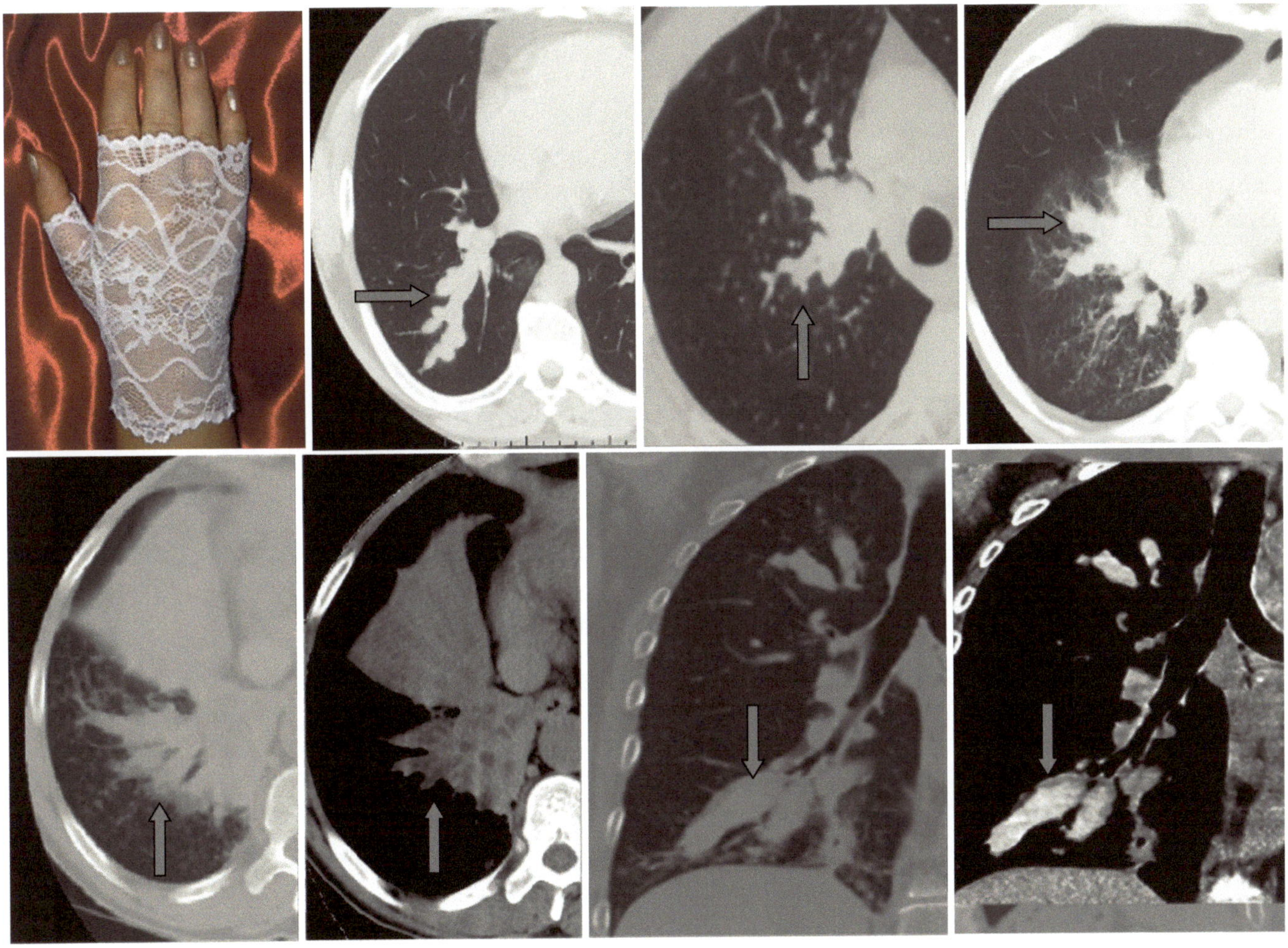

The presence of central bronchiectasias in patients with bronchial asthma should suggest to a radiologist allergic bronchopulmonary aspergillosis. In some patients, bronchiectasias are filled with fungal micelle or mucous impactions which form the "*fingers in a glove*" sign (↑). In 25 % of patients, contents of bronchiectasias have high density as the fungus accumulates calcium oxalate. Additional criteria for proper diagnosis are antibodies to *Aspergillae*, high level of *IgE*, and the positive dermal test for fungal antigens. Less often similar changes can be observed in endobronchial growth of a tumor in the central bronchus.

A. Yudin, *Metaphorical Signs in Computed Tomography of Chest and Abdomen*,
DOI 10.1007/978-3-319-04013-4_27, © Springer International Publishing Switzerland 2014

Atoll or Reversed Halo Sign

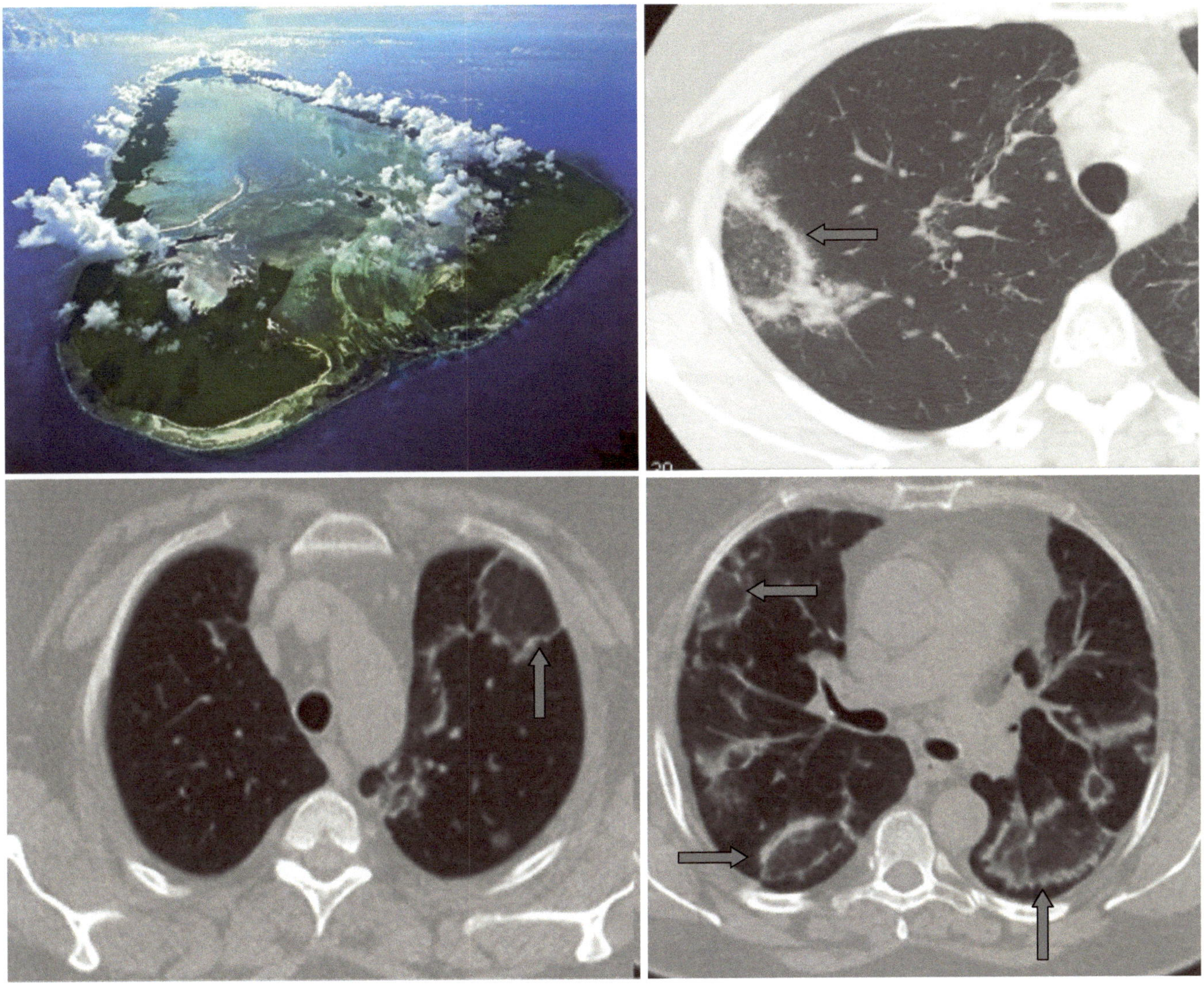

Roundish or crescent stripes and bands of consolidation surrounding zones of ground-glass attenuation in the lungs form the "*atoll*" or "*reversed halo*" sign (↑). Contours are usually rough. This appearance corresponds to the manifestation of a variant of organizing pneumonia.

A. Yudin, *Metaphorical Signs in Computed Tomography of Chest and Abdomen*,
DOI 10.1007/978-3-319-04013-4_28,

Parachute Sign

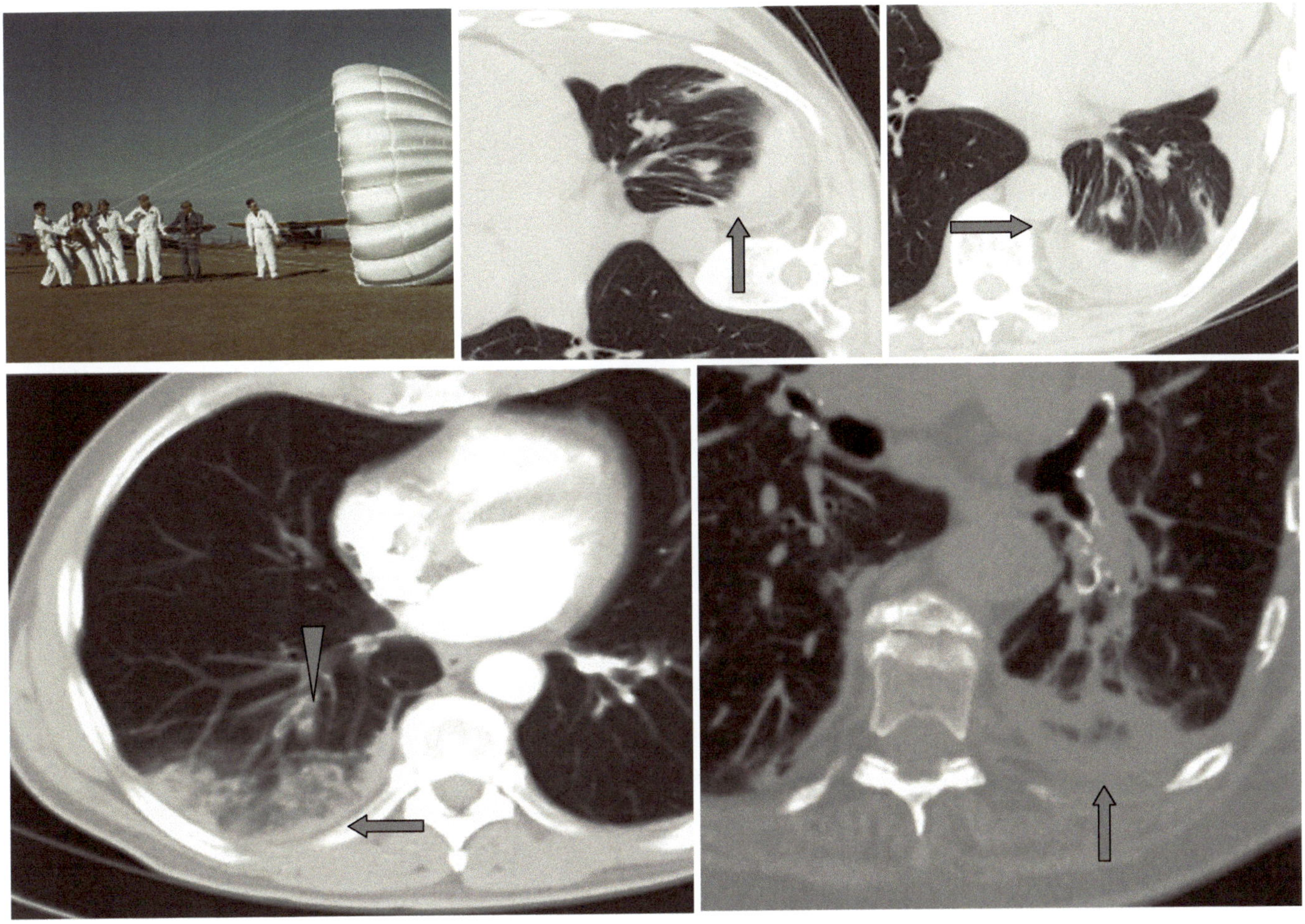

The "*parachute*" sign (↑) is one of the variants of demonstration of infarct pneumonia after pulmonary artery thromboembolism (also the Hampton's hump sign is widely known). The subpleural zone of consolidation in the form of a parachute dome has a higher density at the periphery, and the central part can contain pseudocavitations. Widened "neogenic" vessels extend from the lung hilum to the zone of consolidation forming parachute straps. At CT angiopulmonography thrombi can be detected (Δ) in the pulmonary artery branches corresponding to consolidation.

A. Yudin, *Metaphorical Signs in Computed Tomography of Chest and Abdomen*,
DOI 10.1007/978-3-319-04013-4_29, © Springer International Publishing Switzerland 2014

Atelectasis Discoidea, Atelectasis Lamellosa, or Platelike Atelectasis

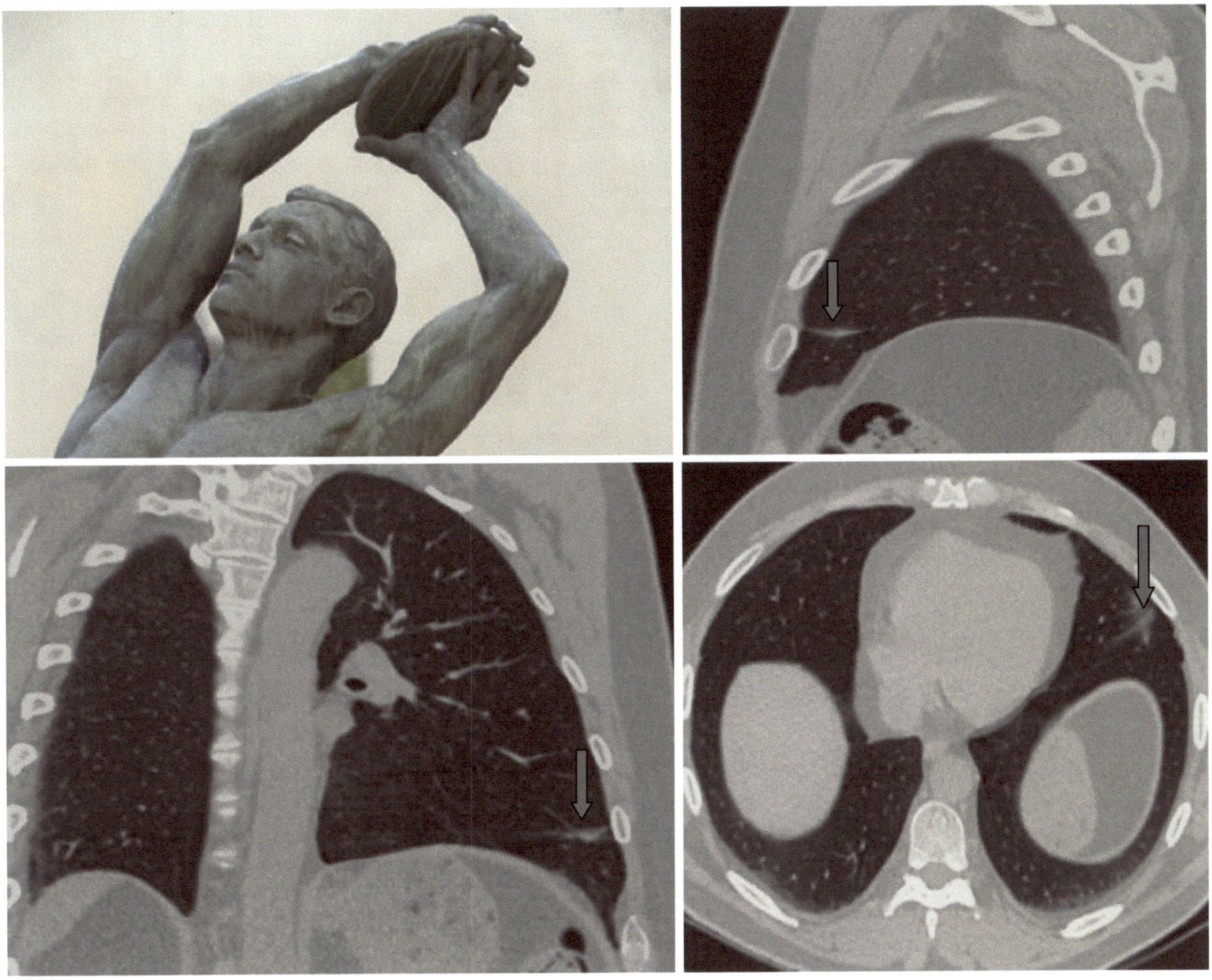

Atelectasis in the form of a disk or a plate (striate, lamellar) – *atelectasis discoidea, atelectasis lamellosa, or platelike atelectasis* (↑) – can develop under pulmonary circulation congestion and hypoventilation, including that caused by low diaphragm excursion in acute diseases of abdominal organs (pancreatitis, peritonitis, perforated stomach ulcer, diseases of the liver and bile ducts).

A. Yudin, *Metaphorical Signs in Computed Tomography of Chest and Abdomen*,
DOI 10.1007/978-3-319-04013-4_30, © Springer International Publishing Switzerland 2014

Mesa, Tafelberg, or Table Mountain Sign

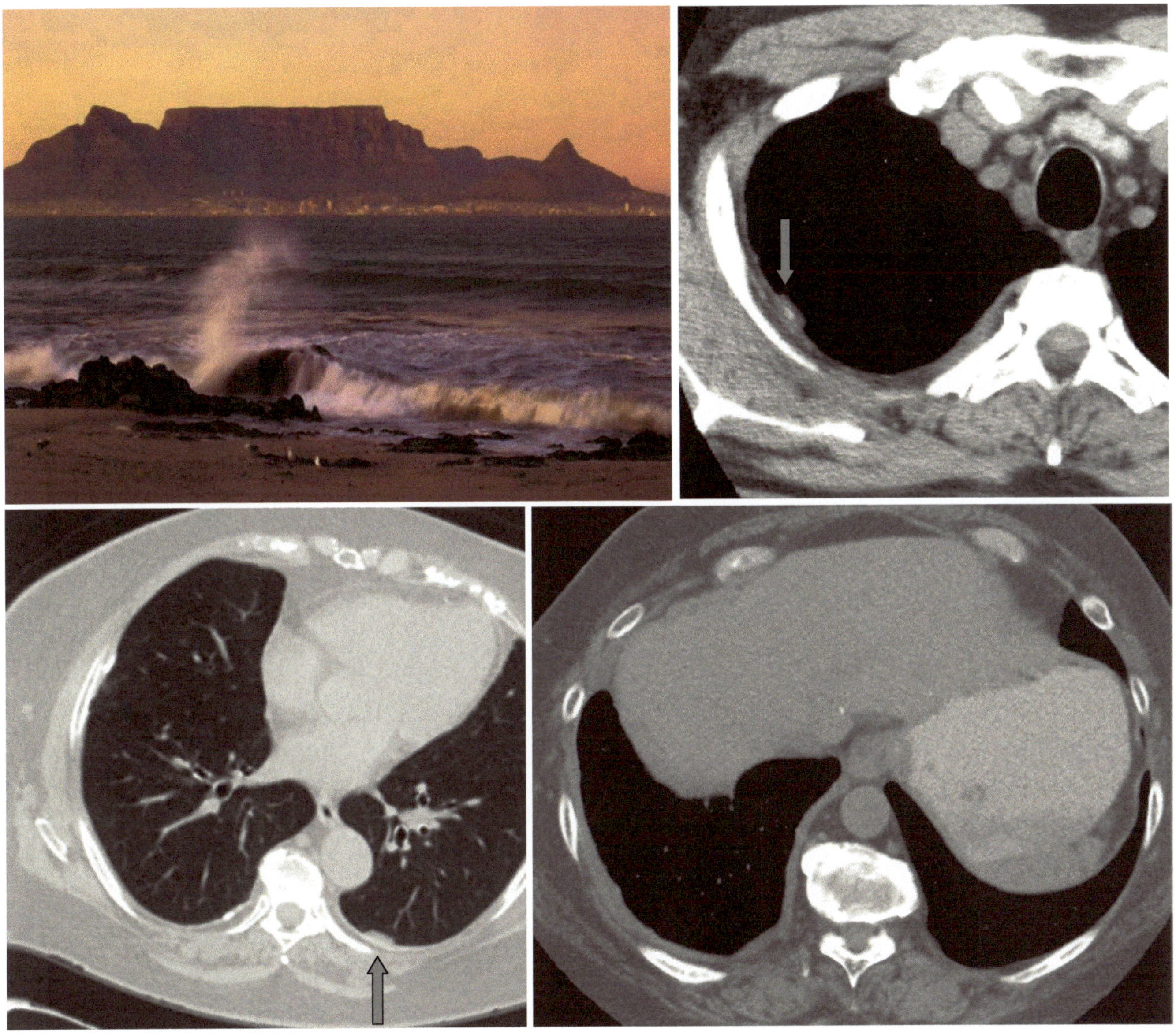

Mesa is a flat-topped mountain to the southwest of Cape Town.

The pleural disease caused by asbestosis can manifest itself in occurrence of pleural plaques, effusion, and diffuse pleural thickening. Pleural plaques consist of fibrous tissue, contain asbestos fibers, frequently calcify in the central part, and on images have "square shoulders" resembling a flat mountain – the "mesa," "*tafelberg*," or "*table mountain*" sign (↑). Diffuse pleural thickening can be found in 5 % of patients with asbestosis that usually is a consequence of benign pleural effusion (right lower image).

A. Yudin, *Metaphorical Signs in Computed Tomography of Chest and Abdomen*,
DOI 10.1007/978-3-319-04013-4_31, © Springer International Publishing Switzerland 2014

Pleural Mouse, Fibrin Body, Fibrin Ball, and Thoracolith

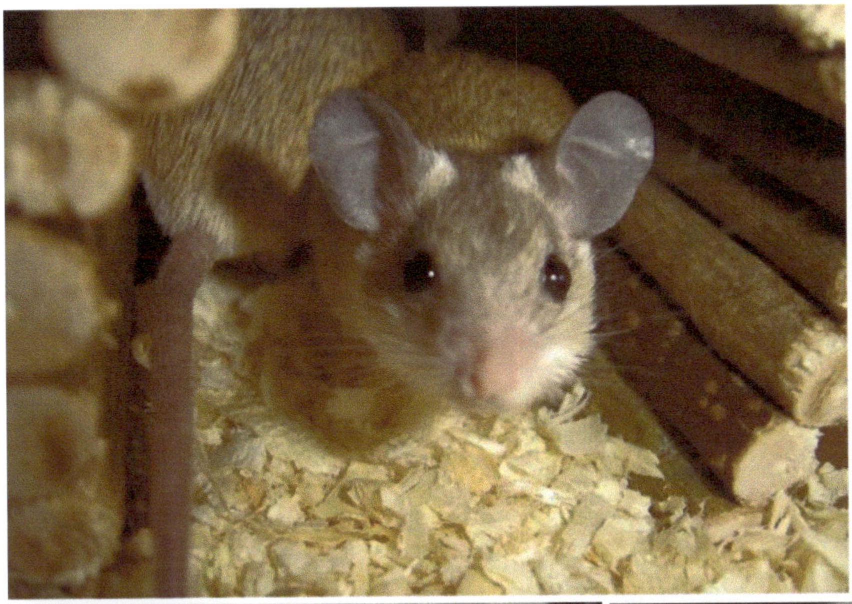

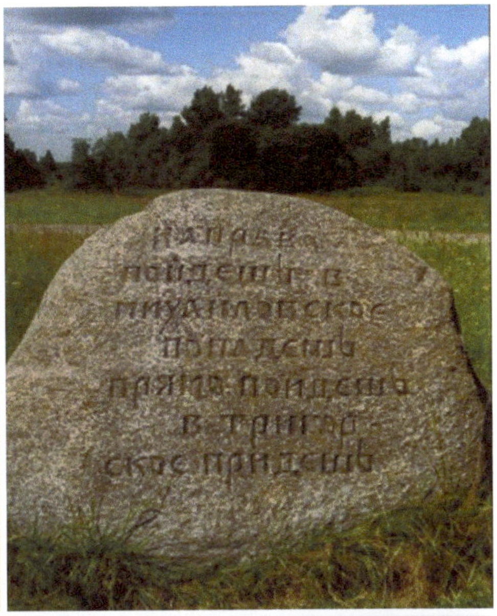

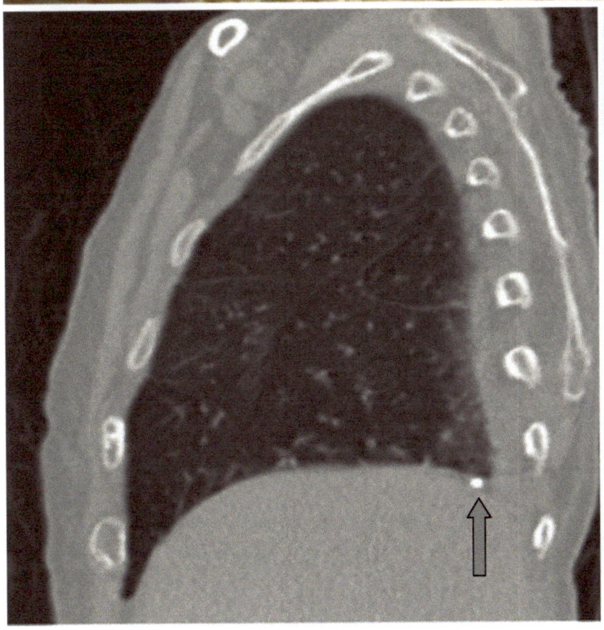

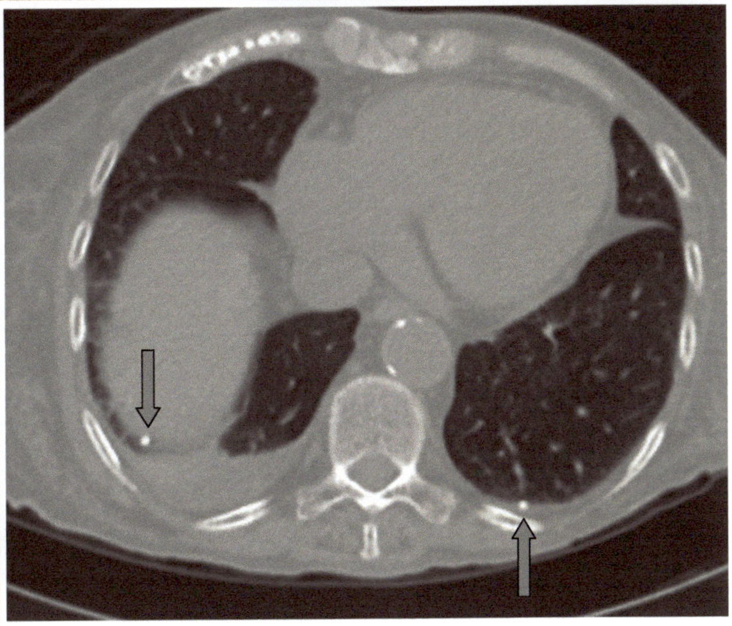

A fibrin clot in the pleural cavity ("*fibrin body*", "*fibrin ball*", or "*pleural mouse*") can be formed in the resolution process of exudative effusion or hemothorax – a soft tissue globule up to 2 cm in diameter. On CT this globule contacts the pleural surface and can spontaneously shift after a change of the patient's position or at a repeat imaging. The fibrin body can exist for a long time, resolve, or calcify turning into a *thoracolith* (↑).

A. Yudin, *Metaphorical Signs in Computed Tomography of Chest and Abdomen*,
DOI 10.1007/978-3-319-04013-4_32, © Springer International Publishing Switzerland 2014

Draped Aorta Sign

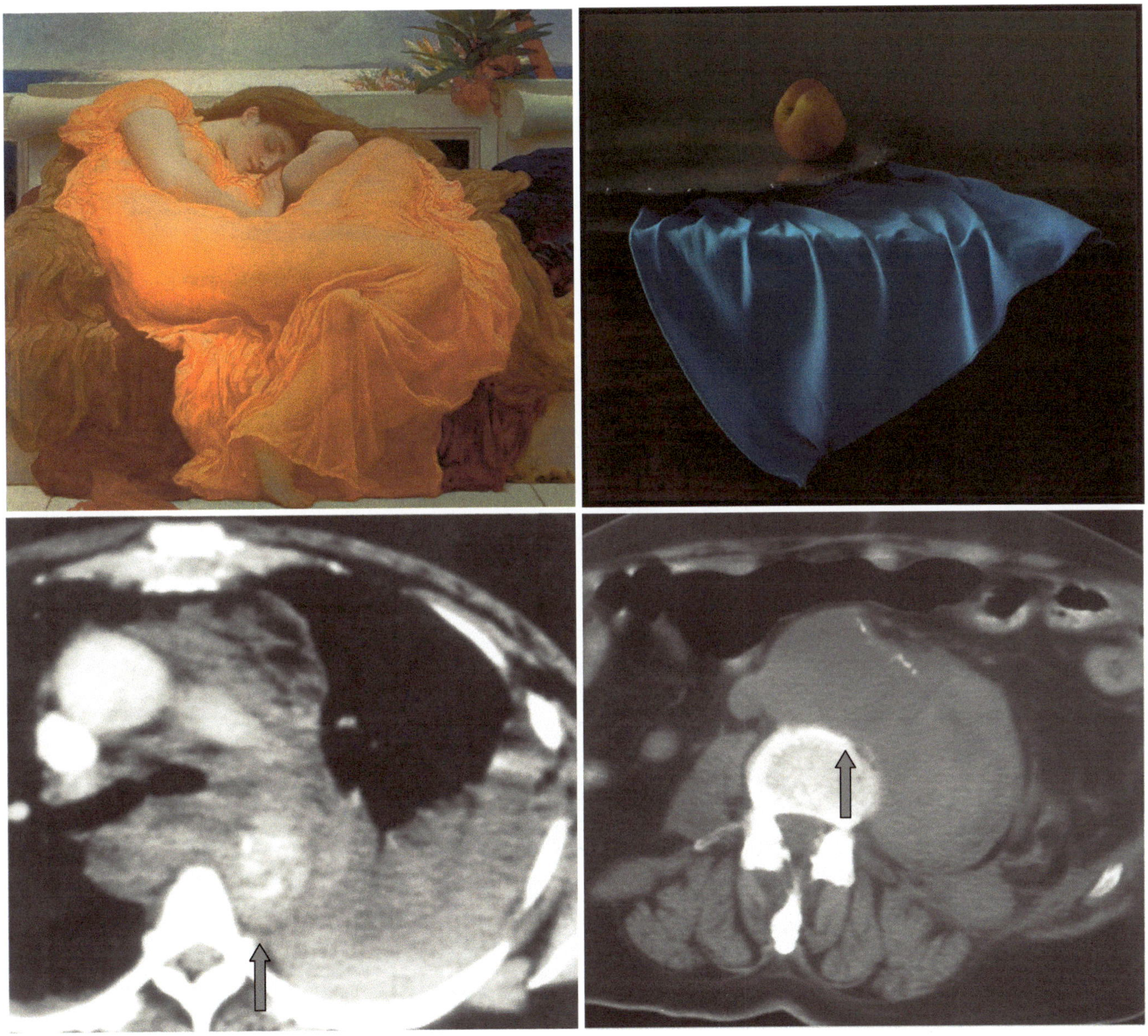

The "*draped aorta*" sign (↑) can indicate a recent rupture of the aorta. This sign manifests itself as a blurred aortic back wall or its wide intimate contact with the contour of the vertebral body. Such signs as "hematocrit," "sentinel clot," and "hyperdense crescent" can also be visible.

A. Yudin, *Metaphorical Signs in Computed Tomography of Chest and Abdomen*,
DOI 10.1007/978-3-319-04013-4_33, © Springer International Publishing Switzerland 2014

Sentinel Clot Sign

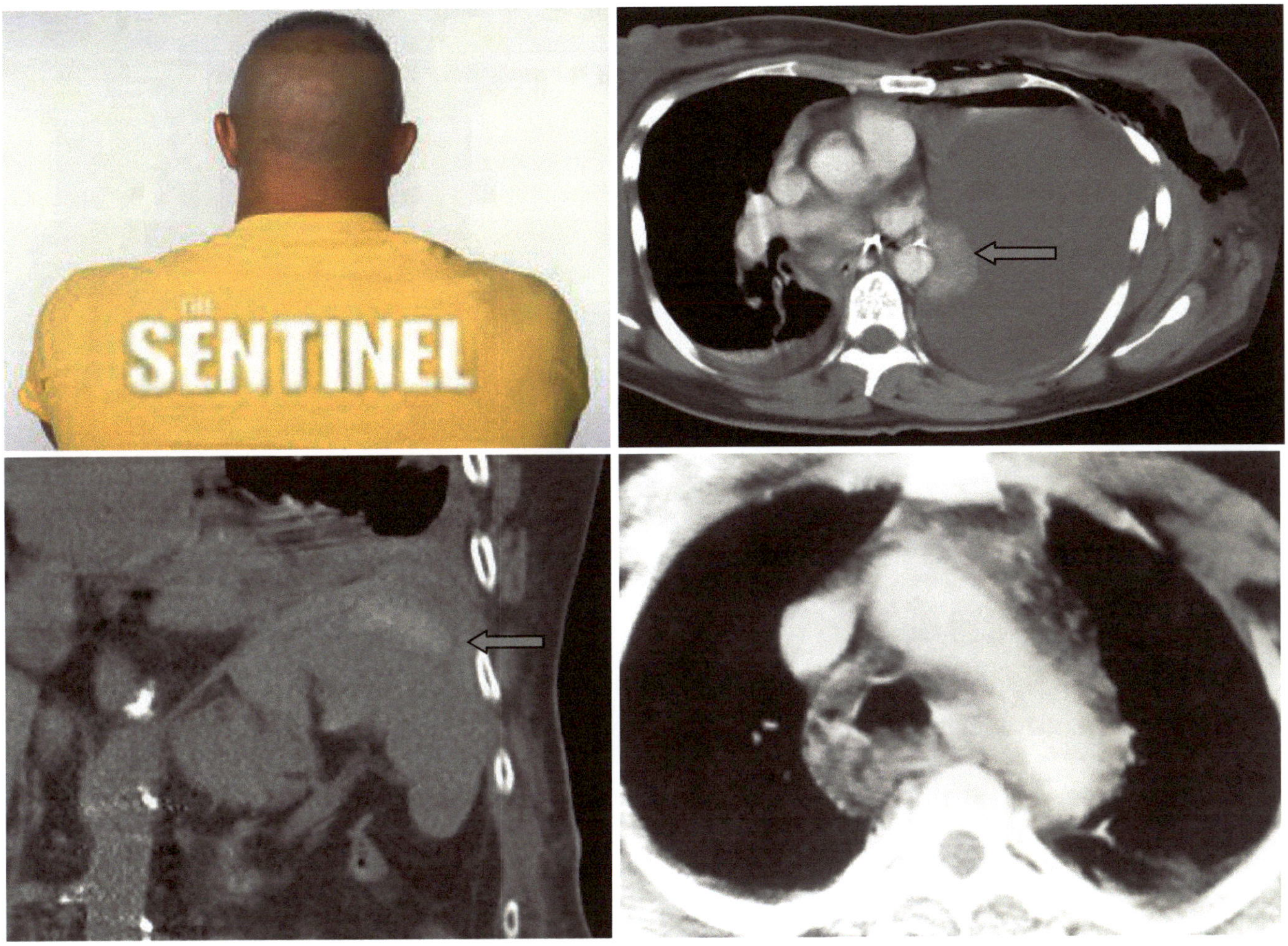

A restricted area of high density near any organ or vessel found after a trauma or surgery represents a hematoma "covering" the zone of rupture – the "*sentinel clot*" sign (↑). This sign points to a trauma (rupture) even in the absence of visible signs of damage to an organ or a vessel. Most obviously the sign is visible at native study and can be missed on enhanced CT (the right lower image).

A. Yudin, *Metaphorical Signs in Computed Tomography of Chest and Abdomen*,
DOI 10.1007/978-3-319-04013-4_34, © Springer International Publishing Switzerland 2014

Intimal Flap and Beak Sign

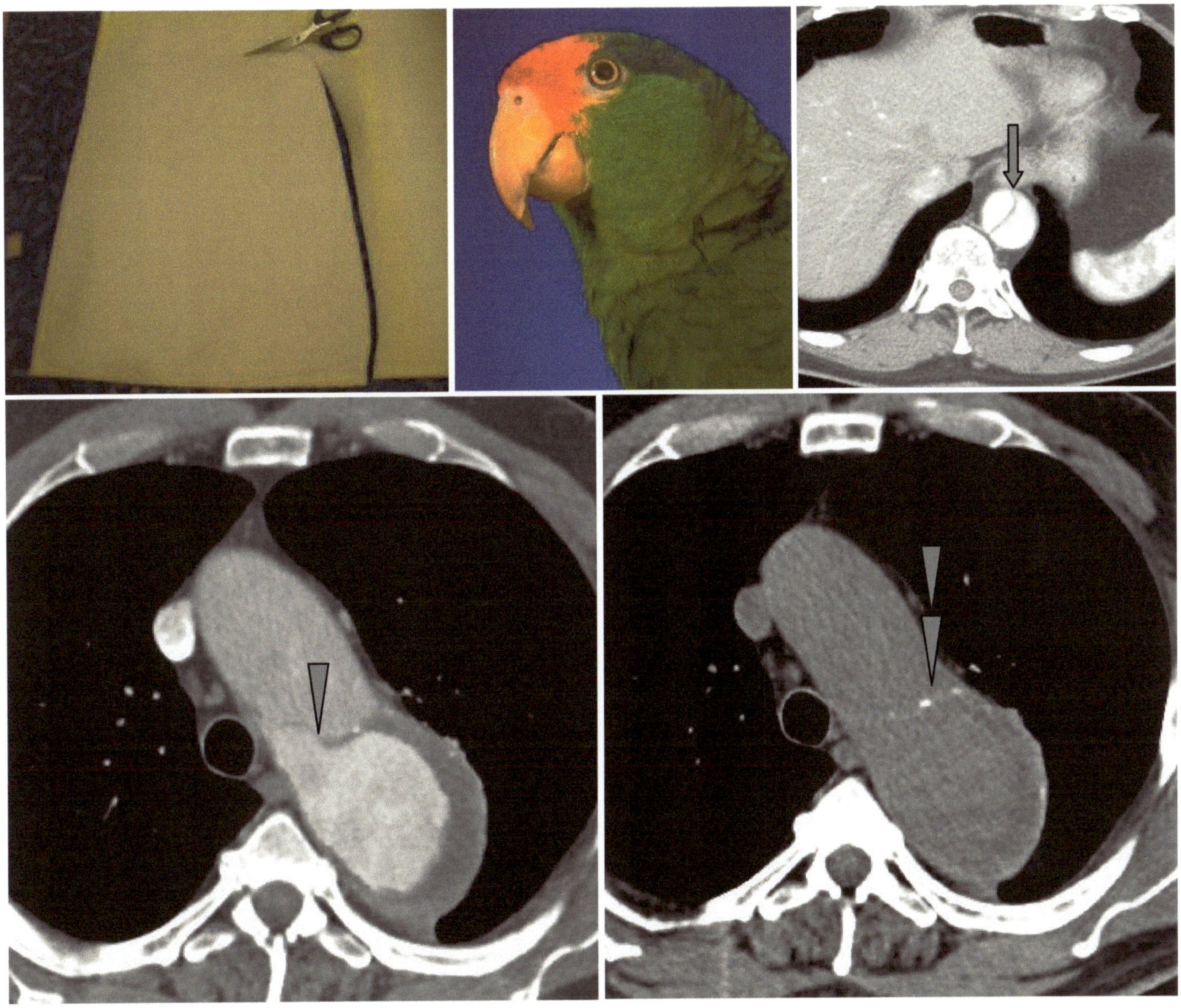

Detection of an "*intimal flap*" (better intimomedial flap) must be considered as the most reliable sign of aortic dissection which represents a linear filling defect after IV enhancement (Δ). This flap separates true and false channels of the aorta. The sharp marginal angle between the aortic wall and the intimal flap so as its crescent form – "*beak*" sign – usually indicates the channel with lower intraluminal pressure (↑). These changes in the aorta can coexist with the "cobweb" sign. On native images, the "beak" sign becomes apparent when calcified intima moves inside (►►).

A. Yudin, *Metaphorical Signs in Computed Tomography of Chest and Abdomen*,
DOI 10.1007/978-3-319-04013-4_35, © Springer International Publishing Switzerland 2014

Cobweb Sign and Mercedes-Benz Sign

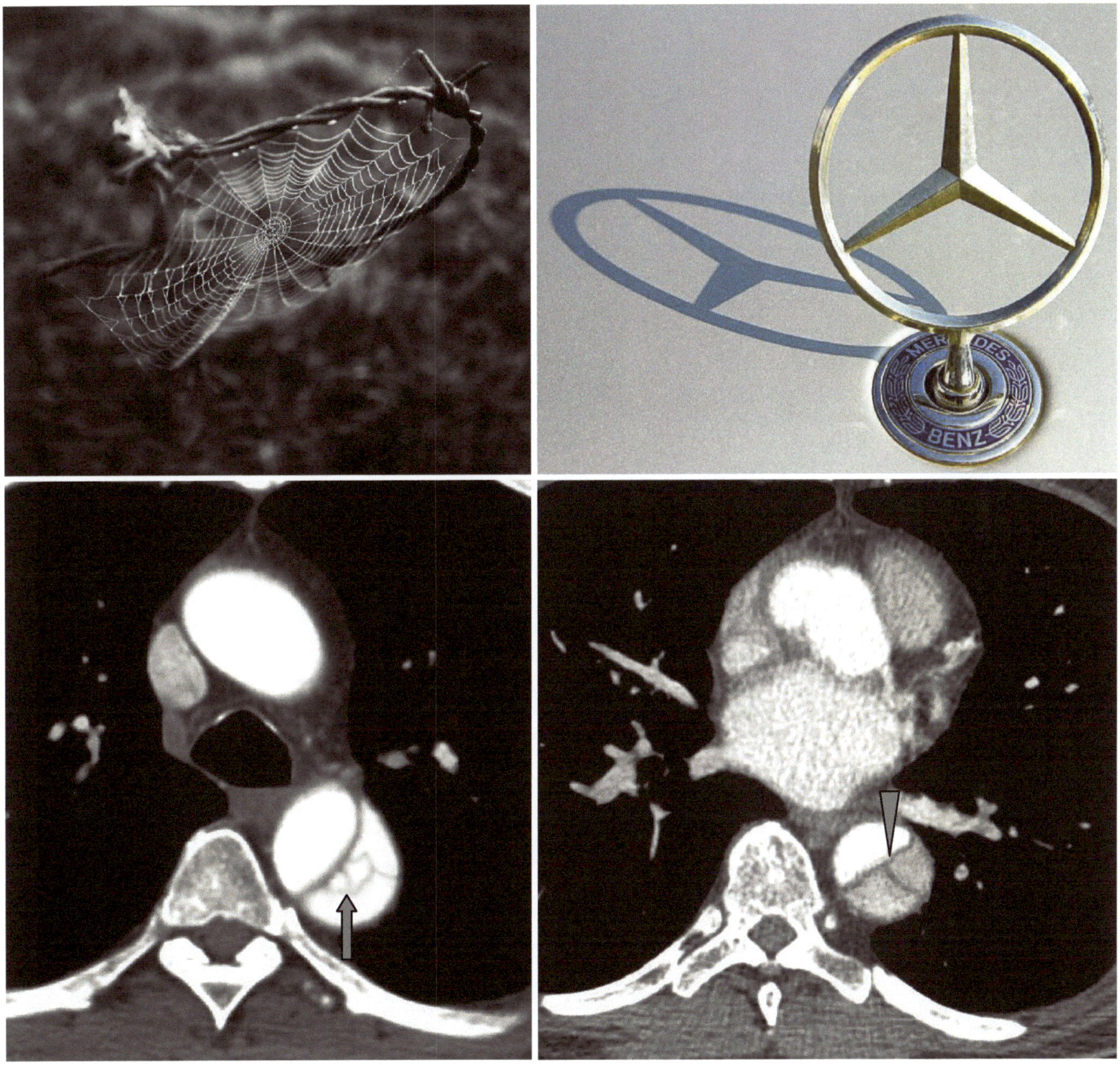

After IV enhancement intimal flaps in the false channel of the dissected aorta may create a view of a network or a web, the "*cobweb*" sign (↑), or a symbol of the Mercedes-Benz company, the "*Mercedes-Benz*" sign (Δ). These signs always coexist with the "beak sign."

A. Yudin, *Metaphorical Signs in Computed Tomography of Chest and Abdomen*,
DOI 10.1007/978-3-319-04013-4_36, © Springer International Publishing Switzerland 2014

Hyperdense Crescent Sign and Beret Sign

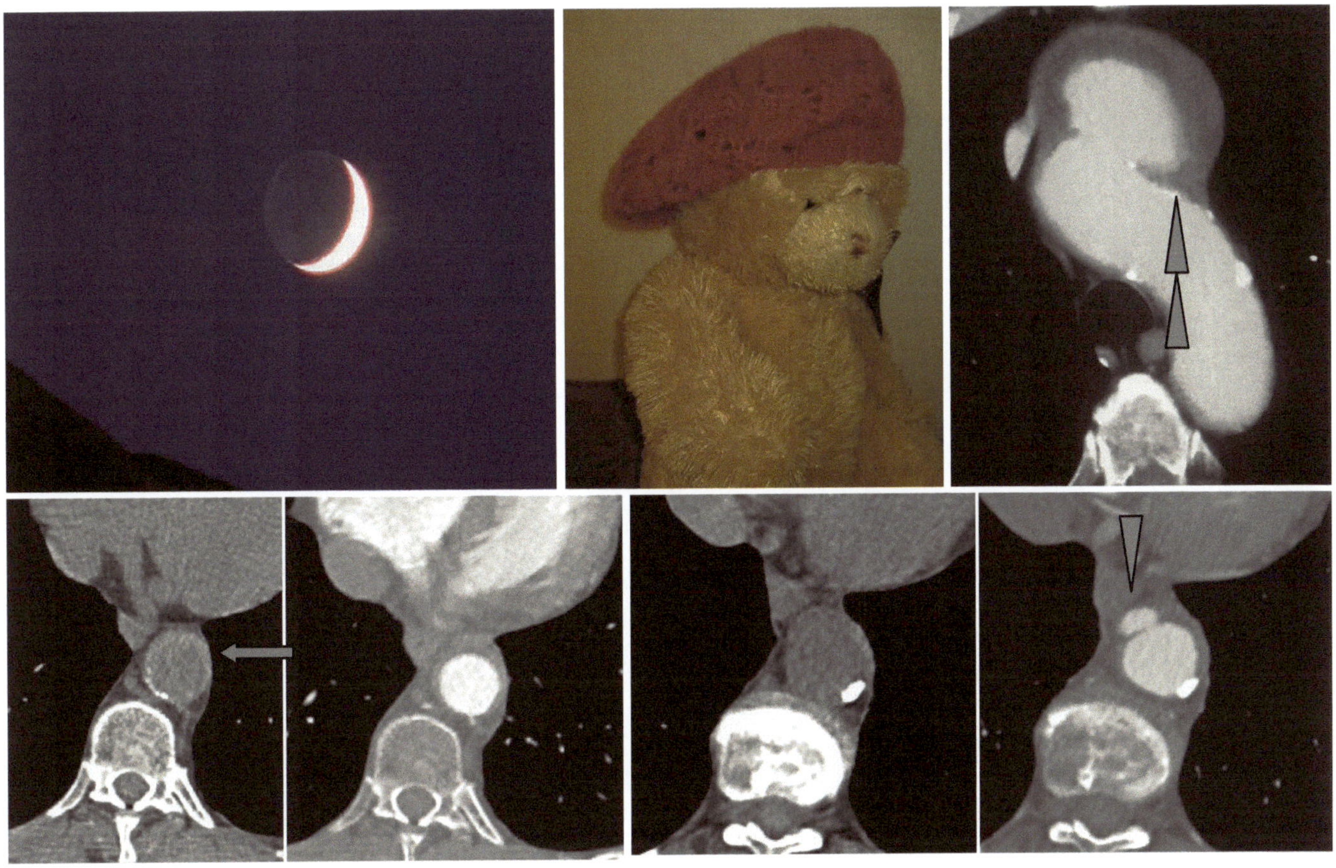

Intramural hematoma caused by trauma or hypertension looks like a hyperdense crescent or a hyperdense ring in a thickened vessel wall on native images – the "*hyperdense crescent*" sign (↑). It is better seen on native images. The penetrating ulcer of the aorta can also be seen as the "hyperdense crescent" sign, but more often after IV enhancement, it represents a local intramural leakage of contrast agent forming the "*beret*" sign (Δ). Intramural hematoma and penetrating ulcer may lead to the formation of a pseudoaneurysm (►►) or dissection.

A. Yudin, *Metaphorical Signs in Computed Tomography of Chest and Abdomen*,
DOI 10.1007/978-3-319-04013-4_37, © Springer International Publishing Switzerland 2014

Web Sign and White (Calcified) Pulmonary Arteries

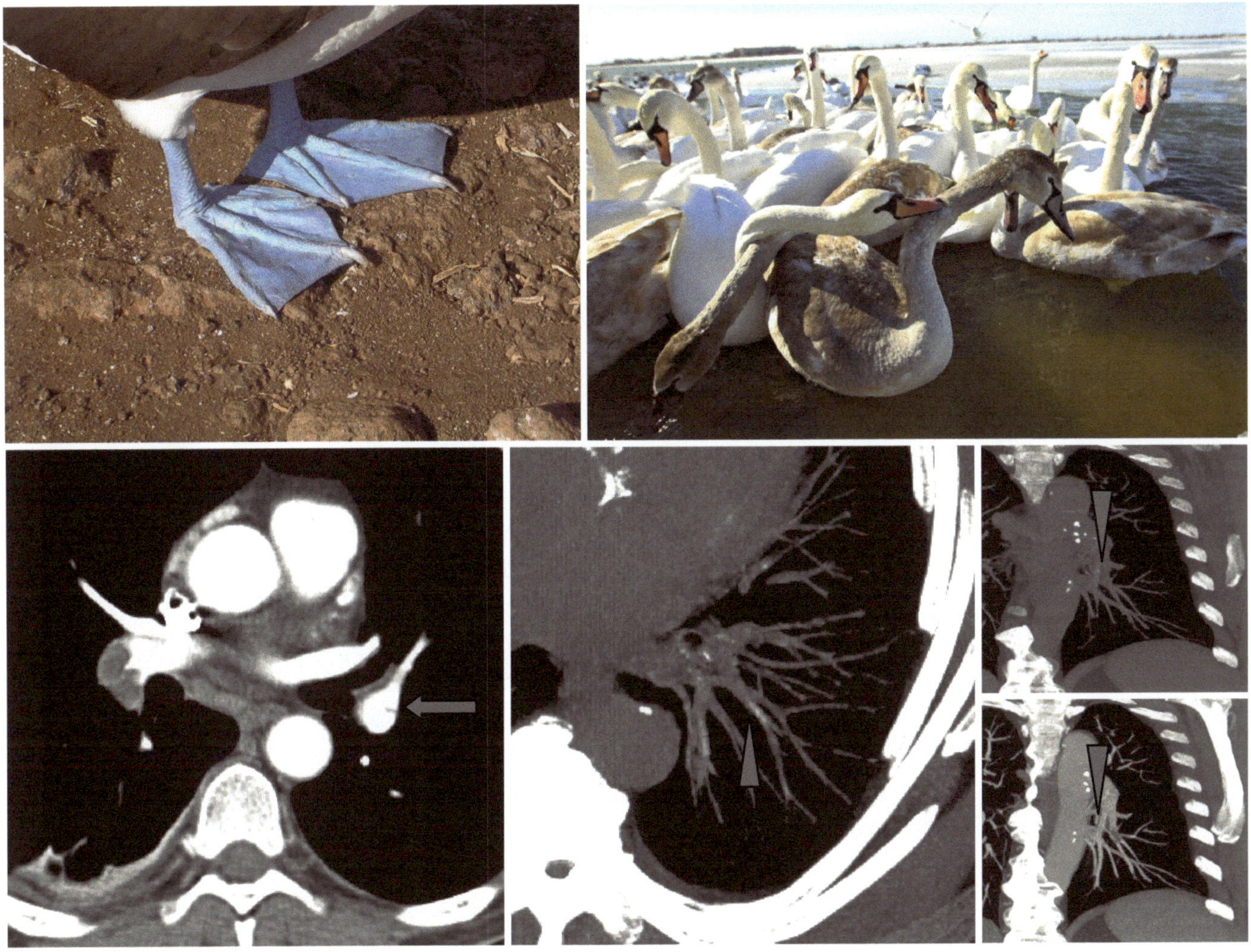

Linear or membrane-filling defects in the pulmonary arteries after IV enhancement must be considered as an additional sign of chronic thromboembolism – the "*web*" sign (↑).

Thrombi in the pulmonary arteries eventually may calcify and look denser (whiter) than normal vessels at native study – "*white or calcified pulmonary arteries*" (Δ). During CT angiopulmonography white sites of the pulmonary arteries can be missed (right lower image).

A. Yudin, *Metaphorical Signs in Computed Tomography of Chest and Abdomen*,
DOI 10.1007/978-3-319-04013-4_38,

Marble Liver Sign or Fatty Liver (Foie Gras)

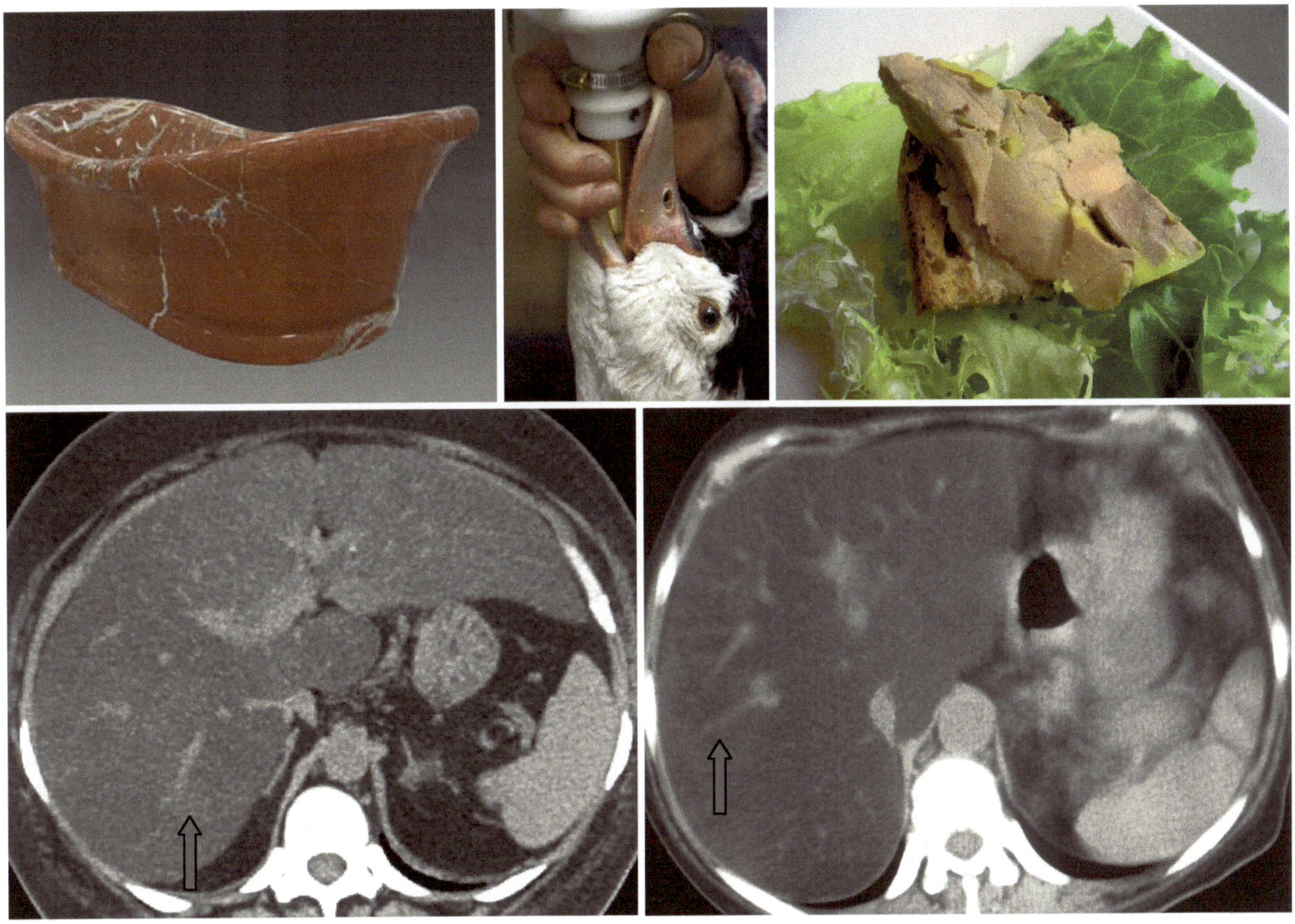

Liver steatosis (fatty liver metamorphosis) is a metabolic complication of a number of toxic, ischemic, and infectious damages to the liver. In steatosis liver density is lower than splenic density. So the vessels without contrast enhancement look hyperdense in comparison with the liver parenchyma forming the "*marble liver*" sign (↑). This sign is also known as "*fatty liver*" that matches *foie gras*.

A. Yudin, *Metaphorical Signs in Computed Tomography of Chest and Abdomen*,
DOI 10.1007/978-3-319-04013-4_39, © Springer International Publishing Switzerland 2014

Geographic Liver

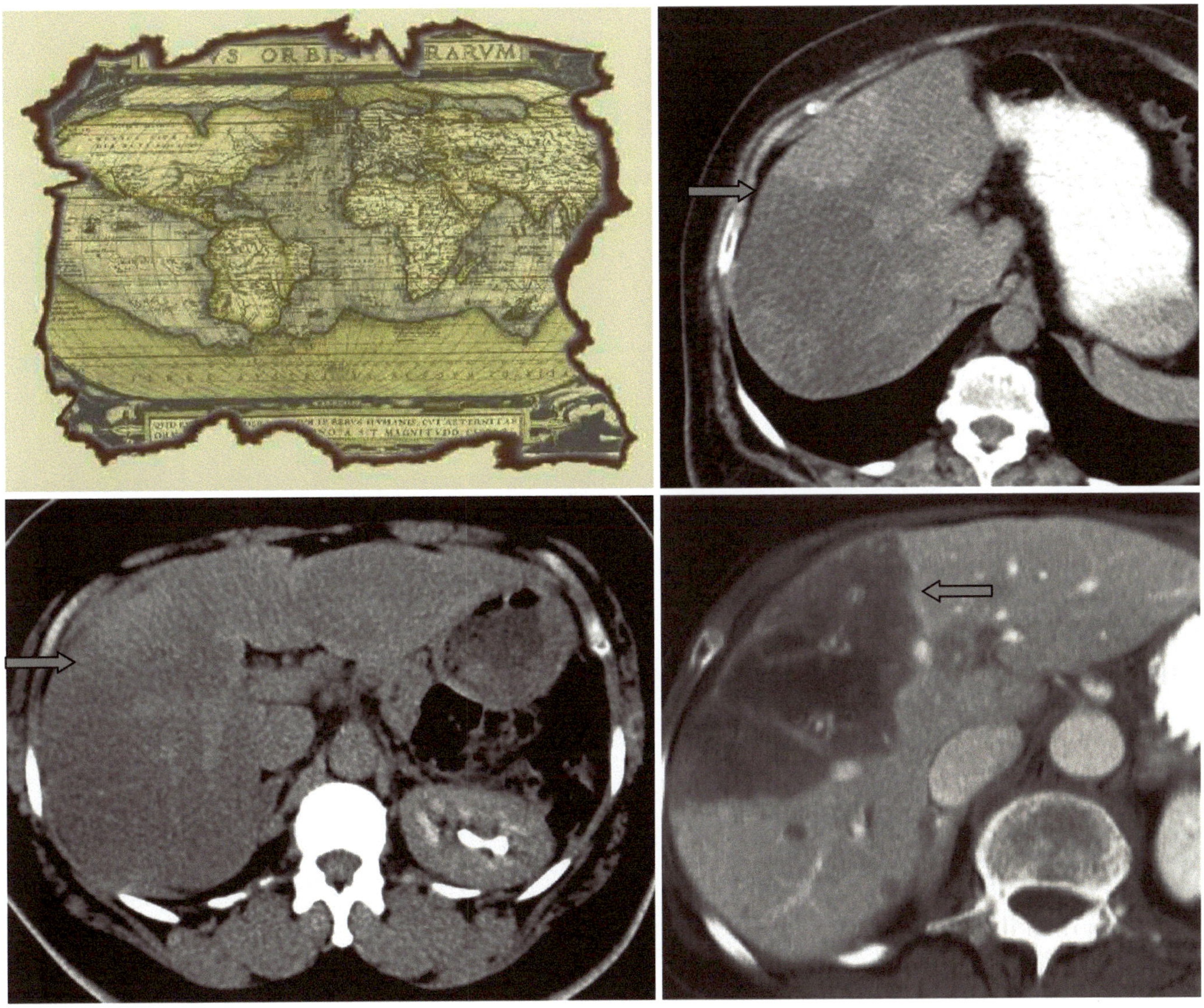

Liver steatosis can be diffuse but also lobar, segmental, and subsegmental. In such cases acute angles and somewhat straight lines of the borders among sites of normal and low densities are distinctly traced – the "*geographic liver*" sign (↑). In the zones with low density, there is no mass effect (vessels do not change normal direction and diameter, and bulging and indrawing of the external liver contour are absent). The presence of steatosis does not guarantee the absence of metastases. Native study must be followed by contrast enhancement.

A. Yudin, *Metaphorical Signs in Computed Tomography of Chest and Abdomen*,
DOI 10.1007/978-3-319-04013-4_40, © Springer International Publishing Switzerland 2014

Boxing Glove Sign

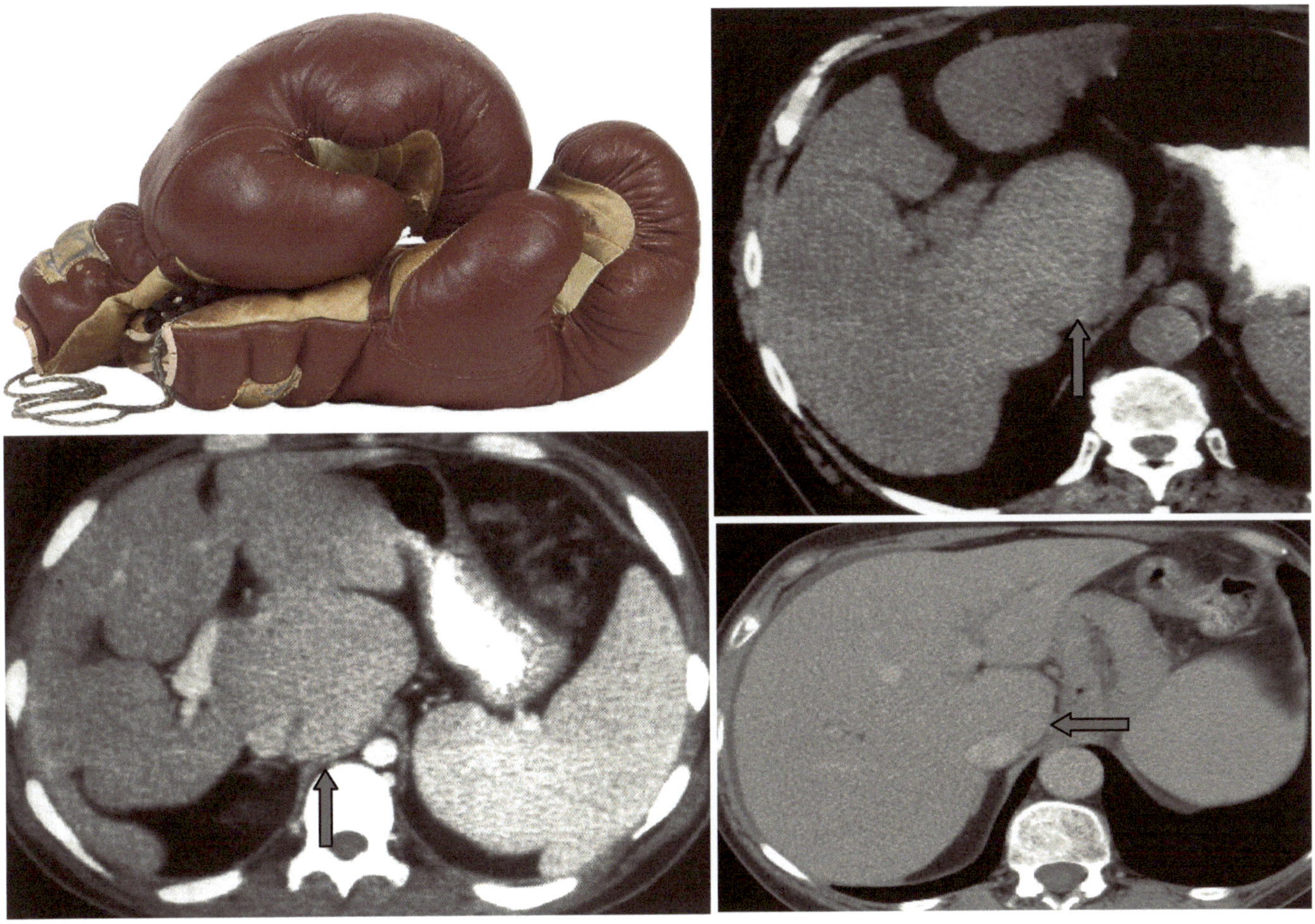

The first liver segment (caudate lobe) that increased in size may be the first and only sign of liver cirrhosis on CT. Covering three borders of the inferior vena cava, the first segment of the liver creates a view of a boxing glove in form – the "*boxing glove*" sign (↑). This sign can be combined with other implications of cirrhosis.

A. Yudin, *Metaphorical Signs in Computed Tomography of Chest and Abdomen*,
DOI 10.1007/978-3-319-04013-4_41, © Springer International Publishing Switzerland 2014

Confluent Fibrosis

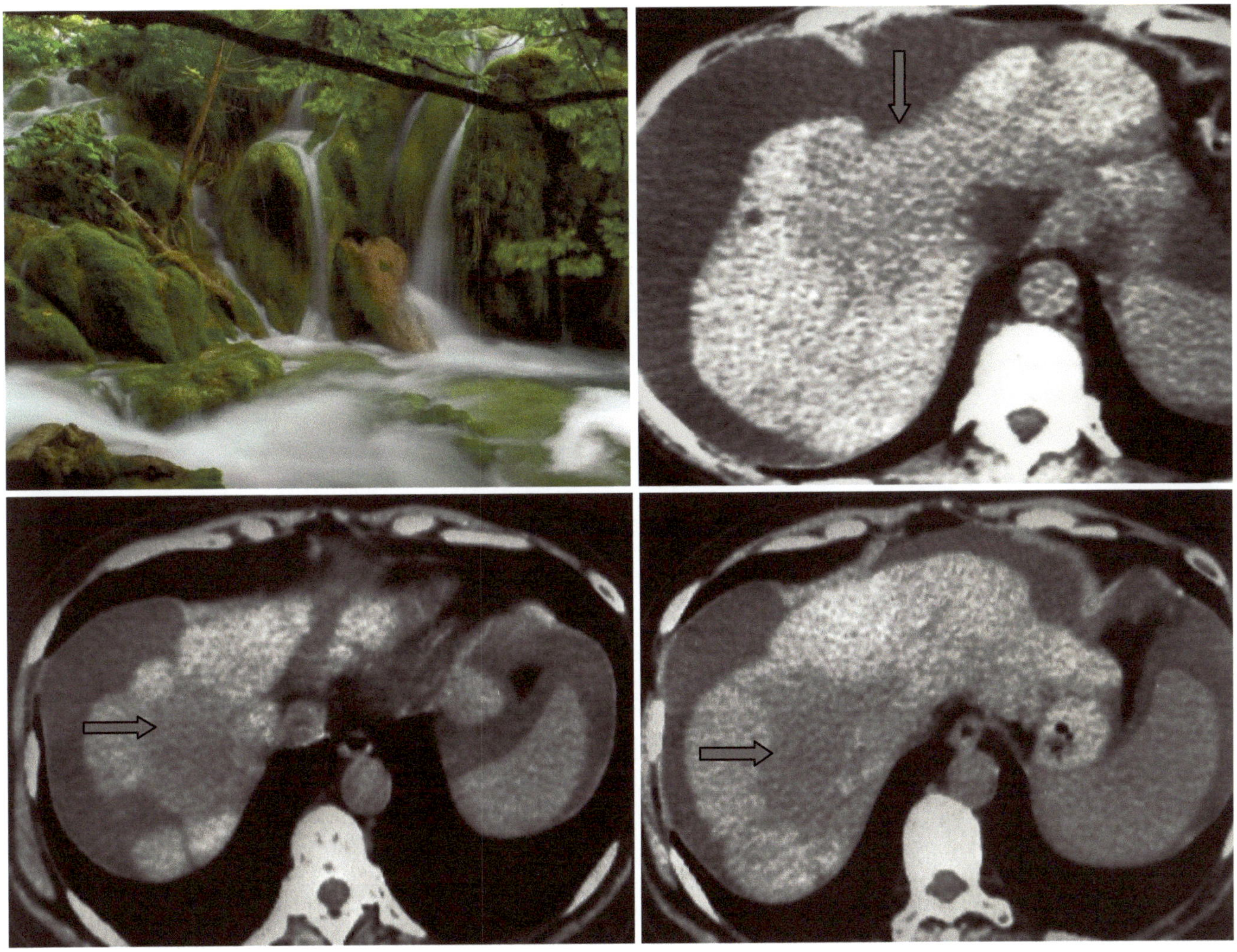

The central liver site of low density with rough and frequently stellate contours is a typical sign of *confluent fibrosis* (↑) in liver cirrhosis. In the parenchymal phase of IV enhancement, the fibrous zone becomes isodense with surrounding parenchyma and less often looks hyperdense. It is possible to find other CT signs of cirrhosis: the "bull's eye," "lacelike or meshy" fibrosis, "salt and pepper," and "white liver."

A. Yudin, *Metaphorical Signs in Computed Tomography of Chest and Abdomen*,
DOI 10.1007/978-3-319-04013-4_42, © Springer International Publishing Switzerland 2014

Bull's Eye Sign

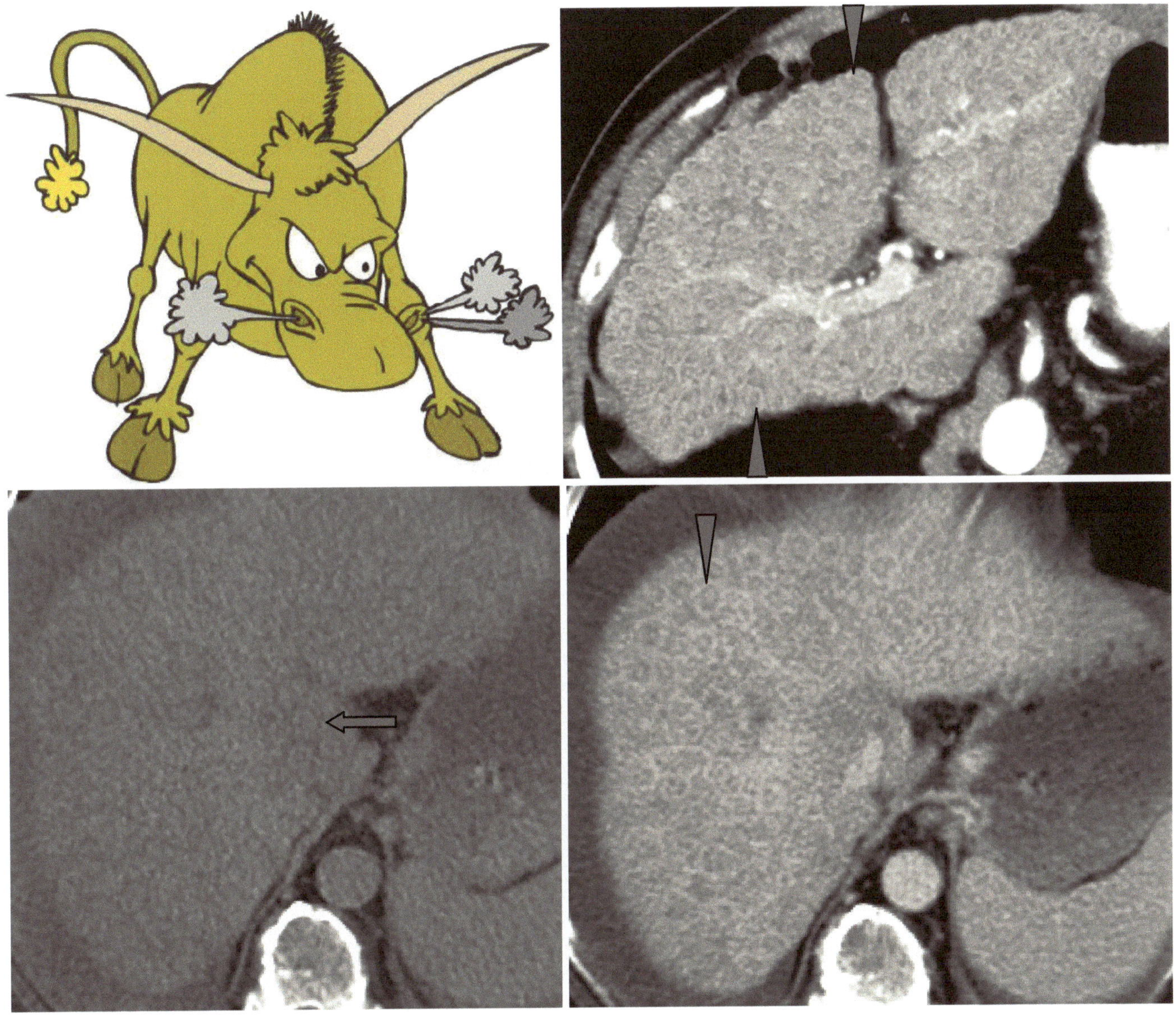

In liver cirrhosis regenerative nodes are surrounded by zones of interstitial fibrosis. The veins pass through the centers of the nodes. On native images node tissue has a higher density than the vessels and interstitium due to the deposition of hemosiderin – the "*reversed bull's eye*" sign (↑). After IV contrast enhancement the veins and fibrous tissue can accumulate contrast agent more intensively than the tissue of regenerative nodes thus forming the "*bull's eye*" sign (Δ). Much more often the densities of the nodes and the fibrous tissue average in parenchymal phase of contrast enhancement.

A. Yudin, *Metaphorical Signs in Computed Tomography of Chest and Abdomen*,
DOI 10.1007/978-3-319-04013-4_43, © Springer International Publishing Switzerland 2014

Lacelike Fibrosis and Salt and Pepper Sign

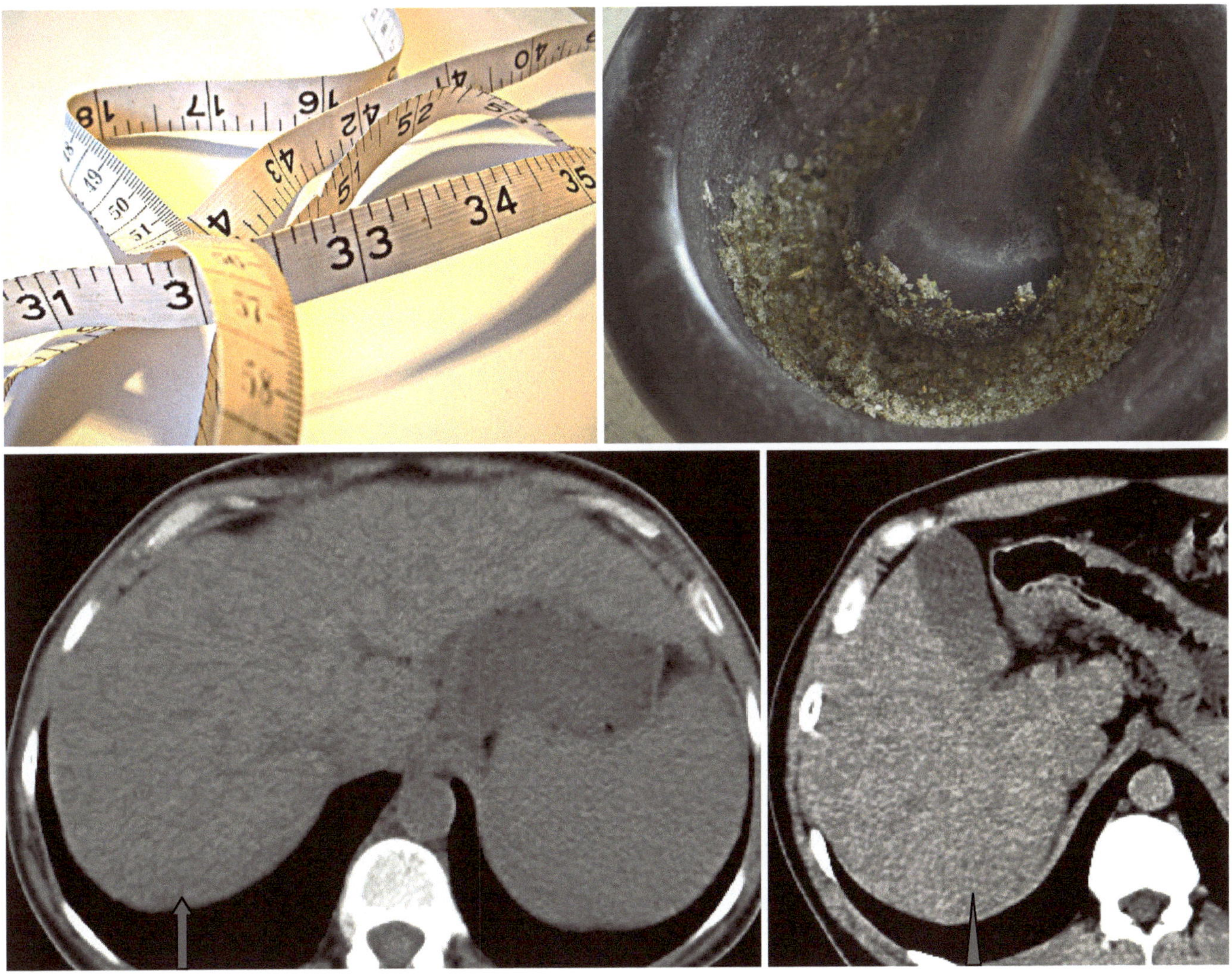

On tomograms the sites of liver interstitial fibrosis can create visual similarity to abundance of hypodense stripes among high-density regenerative nodes forming an image of "*lacelike fibrosis*" (↑). Such fibrosis is also called "*meshy*" and "*reticulated*." If regenerative nodules have a very small size, the "*salt and pepper*" sign (Δ) can be formed – intermittent fine sites of high and low density. Other signs of cirrhosis can also be detected.

A. Yudin, *Metaphorical Signs in Computed Tomography of Chest and Abdomen*,
DOI 10.1007/978-3-319-04013-4_44, © Springer International Publishing Switzerland 2014

White Liver Sign

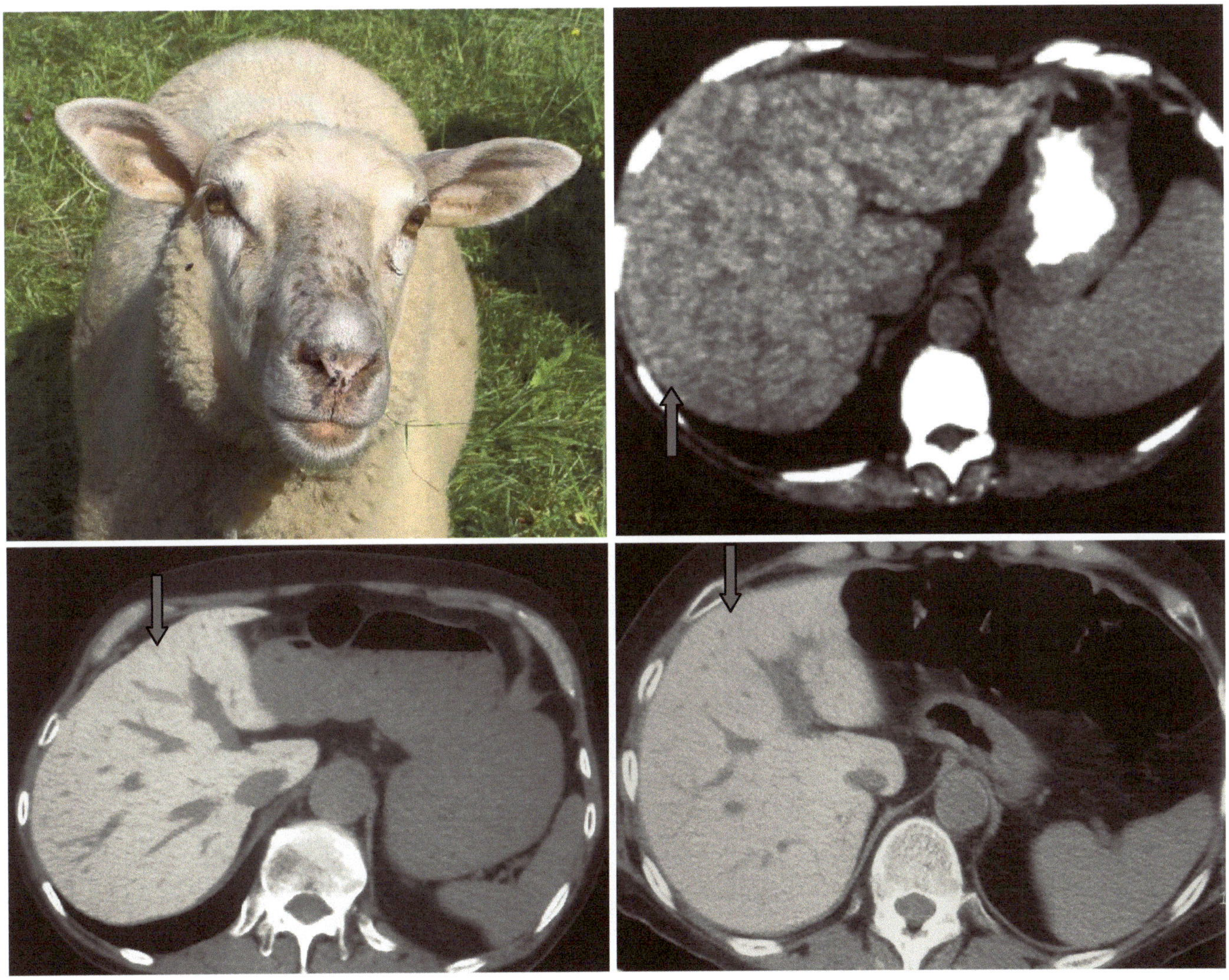

Excess accumulation of substances with high features of X-ray attenuation can lead to a substantial increase in liver density on native images forming the "*white liver*" sign (↑). Most often such changes are visible in cirrhosis because of hemosiderin accumulation in regenerative nodes. High density of the liver can also be found in patients receiving amiodarone as a molecule of this substance includes an atom of iodine.

Do not confuse the CT sign to the disease (white liver disease – visceral steatosis in sheep).

A. Yudin, *Metaphorical Signs in Computed Tomography of Chest and Abdomen*,
DOI 10.1007/978-3-319-04013-4_45, © Springer International Publishing Switzerland 2014

Periportal Halo

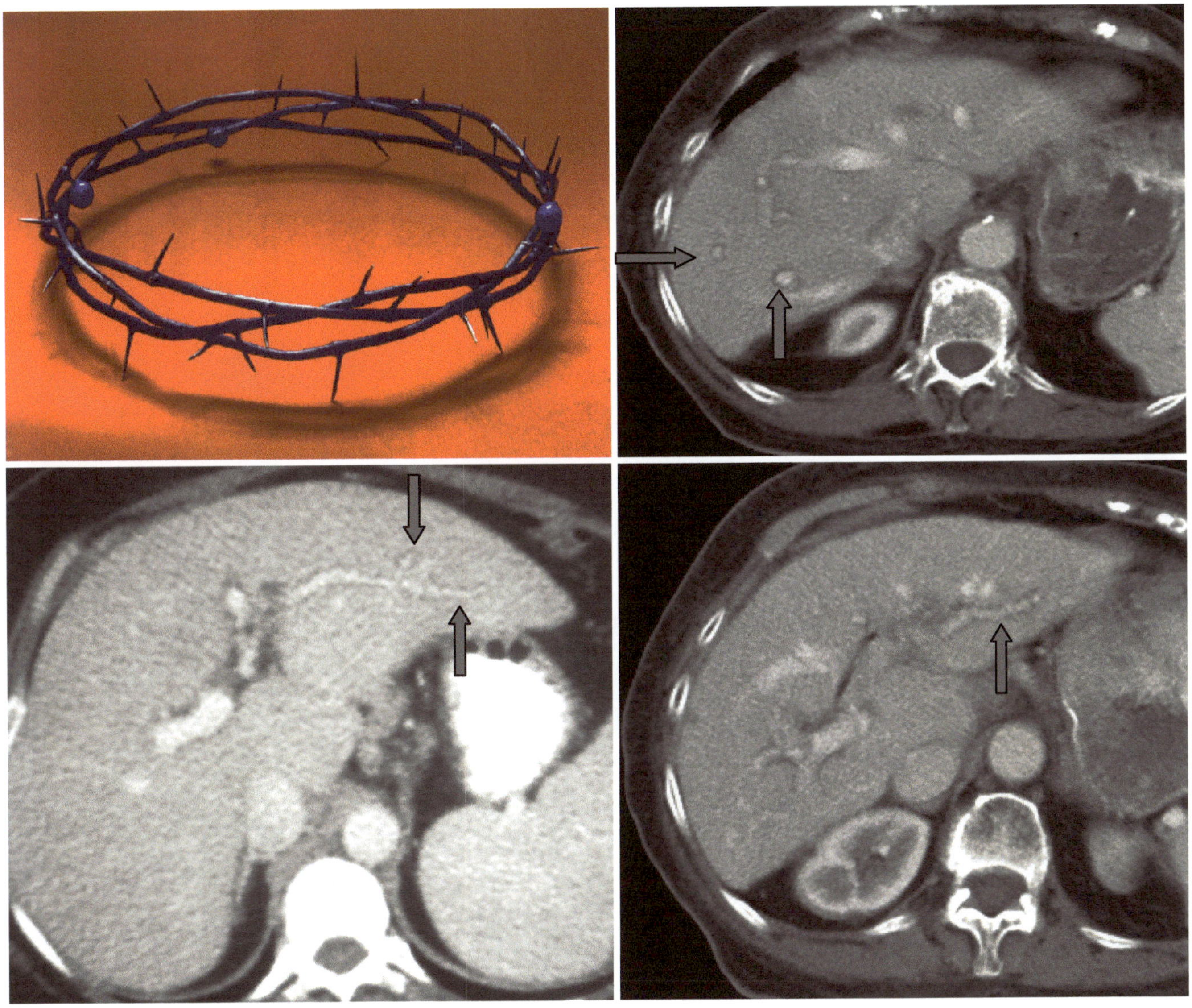

After IV enhancement thin low-density rims around the peripheral branches of the portal vein form the "*periportal halo*" sign (↑) which indicates interstitial edema of the liver. If a branch of the portal vein is located in the tomographic plane, then we speak about the "tram-tracking" sign. The causes of edema can be various: neoplasms and enlarged lymph nodes in the hepatic porta, hepatitis, active phase of autoimmune cirrhosis, congested liver in heart failure, liver trauma, early period after liver transplantation, and others. Do not confuse with biliary ducts dilatation.

A. Yudin, *Metaphorical Signs in Computed Tomography of Chest and Abdomen*,
DOI 10.1007/978-3-319-04013-4_46, © Springer International Publishing Switzerland 2014

Ripples in the Water Sign or Target Sign

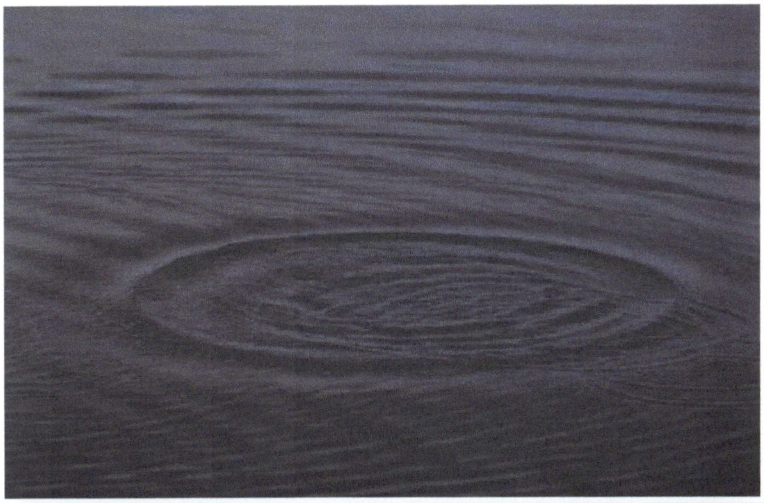

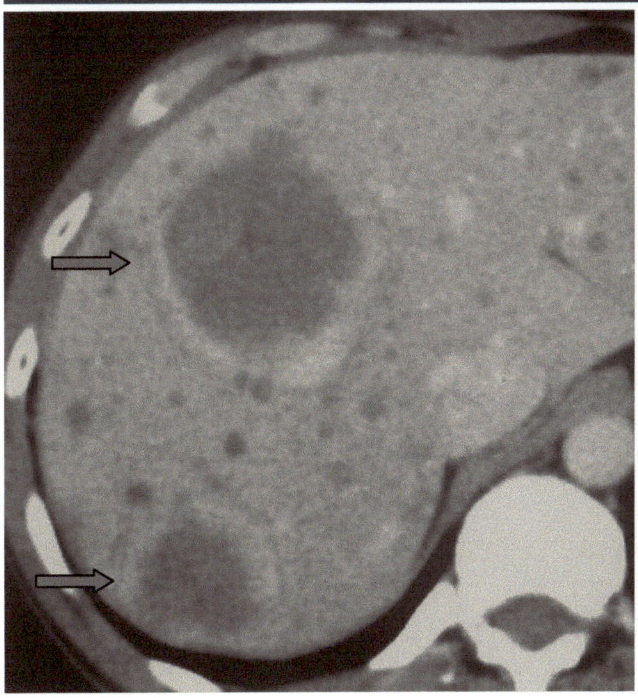

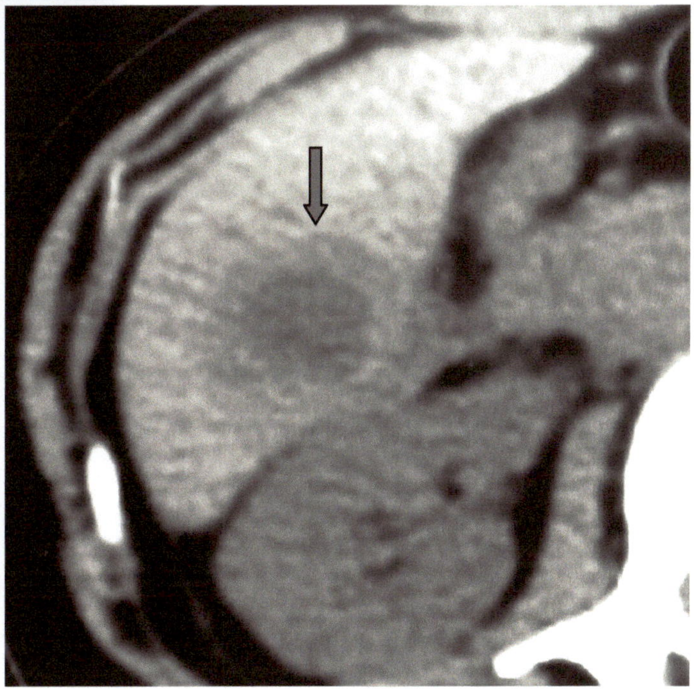

Liver abscess can manifest itself as a hypodense nonuniform formation with a hyperdense capsule (especially after IV contrast enhancement) surrounded by a hypodense zone of edema. This forms the "*ripples in the water*" sign (↑) also known as the "target" sign. This sign may coexist with the "clusters of grapes" sign.

A. Yudin, *Metaphorical Signs in Computed Tomography of Chest and Abdomen*,
DOI 10.1007/978-3-319-04013-4_47, © Springer International Publishing Switzerland 2014

Cluster of Grapes Sign

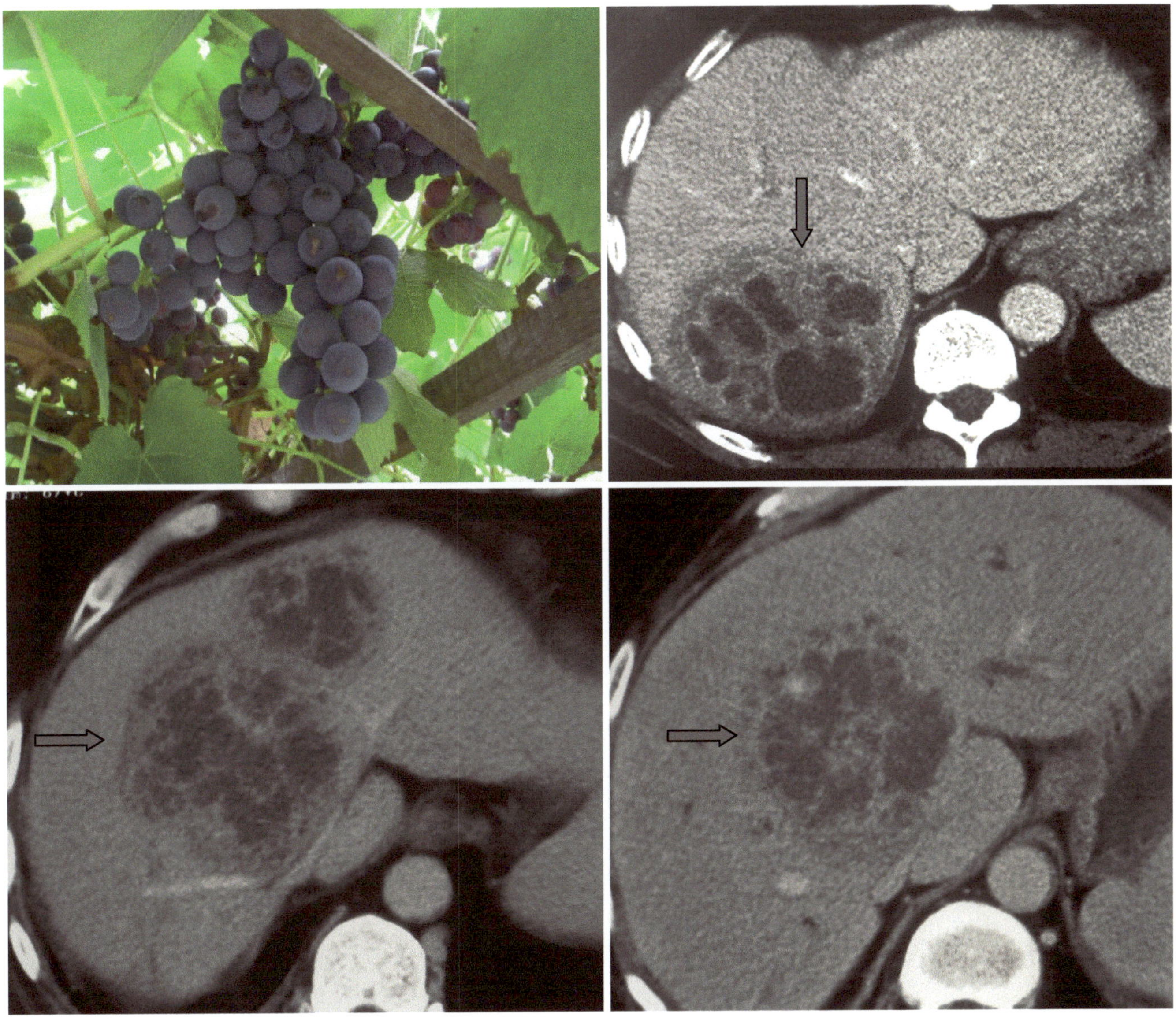

Small pyogenic abscesses of the liver, merging into a large cavity, form an image similar to a bunch of grapes or berries – "*cluster of grapes*" sign (↑). The mature cavity has multiple septa. The density of the cavity contents is a little higher than that of water. The "cluster of grapes" sign can be combined with the "ripples in the water" sign. The presence of gas bubbles is also possible inside abscesses.

A. Yudin, *Metaphorical Signs in Computed Tomography of Chest and Abdomen*,
DOI 10.1007/978-3-319-04013-4_48, © Springer International Publishing Switzerland 2014

Water Lily Sign or Snake Sign

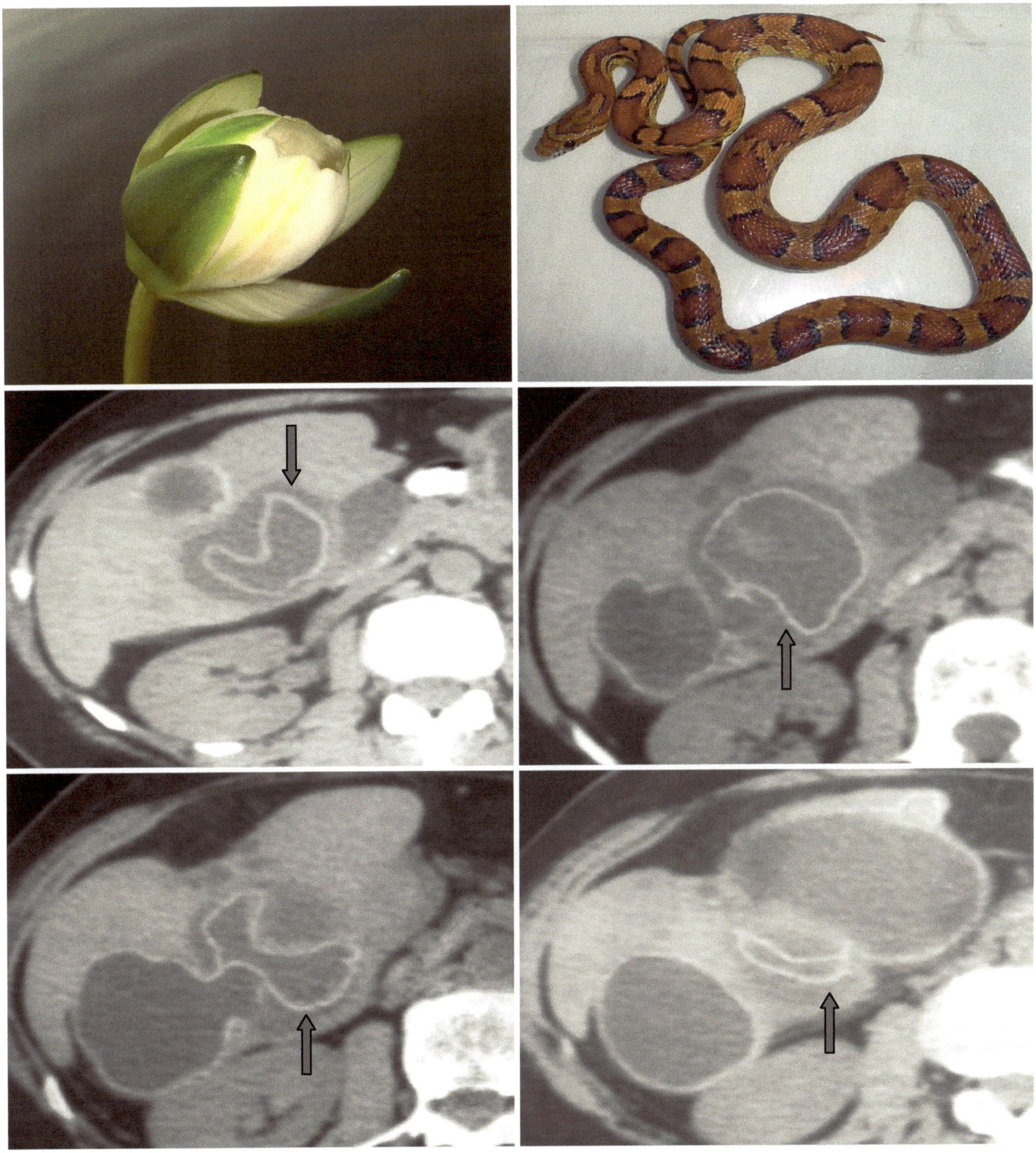

In the course of a hydatid cyst vital activity, the fibrous capsule calcifies and can also peel off (inner pressure in cysts decreases). Free fragments of the capsule in a cyst form the "*water lily*" sign or the "*snake*" sign (↑) which is specific for echinococcosis. Detection of daughter cysts is also a specific sign for *E. granulosus*.

A. Yudin, *Metaphorical Signs in Computed Tomography of Chest and Abdomen*,
DOI 10.1007/978-3-319-04013-4_49,

Bright Dot Sign and Iris or Eye Diaphragm Sign

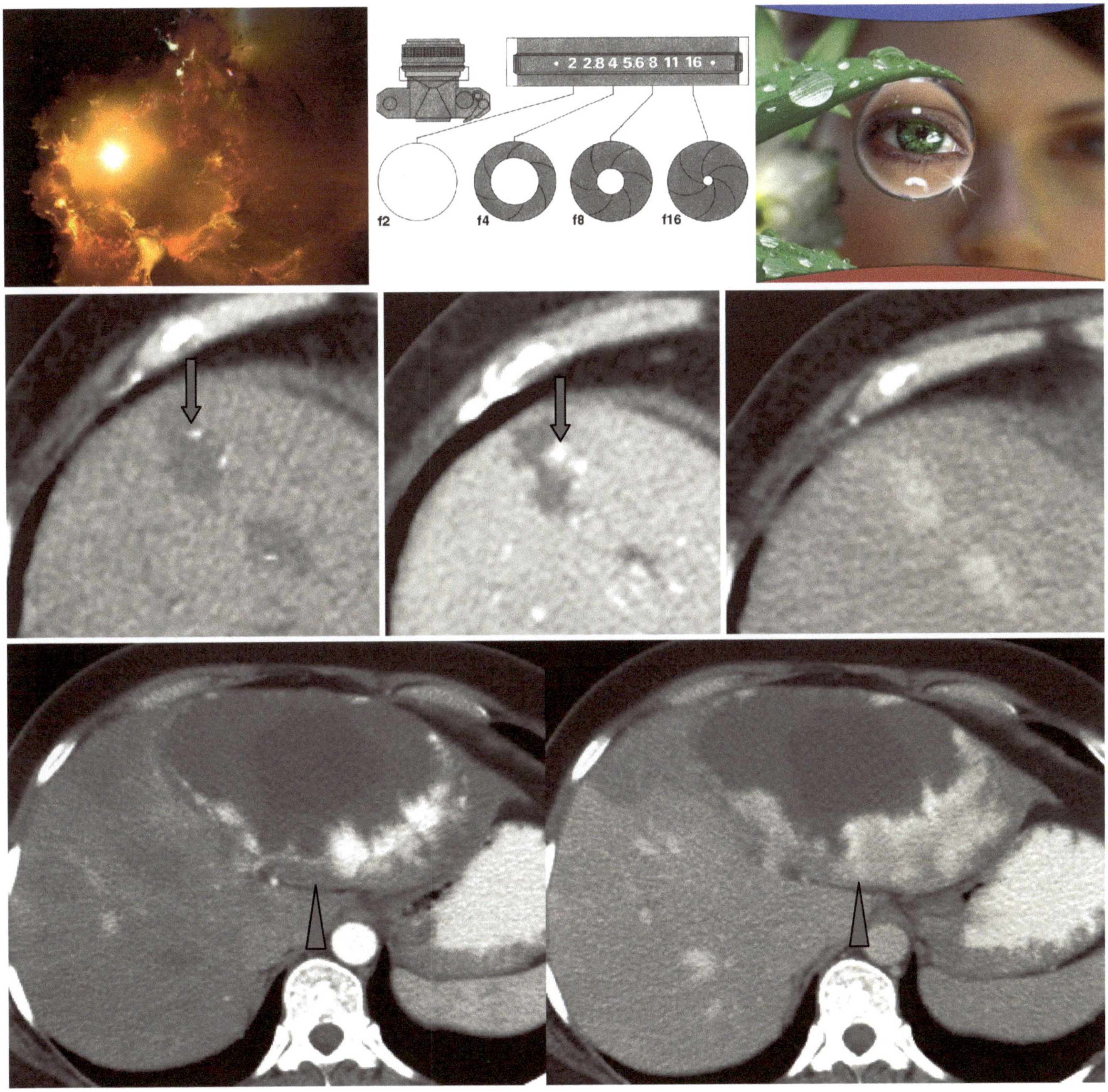

In 80 % of cases, hemangiomas have typical features after IV enhancement. In the arterial phase, foci (lacunas) with high density of blood with contrast agent appear at periphery of the mass – the "*bright dot*" sign (↑). In parenchymal and delayed phases, the foci enlarge in size as the enhanced blood fills lacunar spaces from the periphery to the center.

In all phases of enhancement, lacunas have the density corresponding to density of contrasted vessels (effect of a blood pool). In large hemangiomas centripetal filling of mass with contrast agent is called the "*iris*" sign or the "*eye diaphragm*" sign (Δ).

A. Yudin, *Metaphorical Signs in Computed Tomography of Chest and Abdomen*,
DOI 10.1007/978-3-319-04013-4_50, © Springer International Publishing Switzerland 2014

Stellate Scar Sign or Spoke-Wheel Pattern

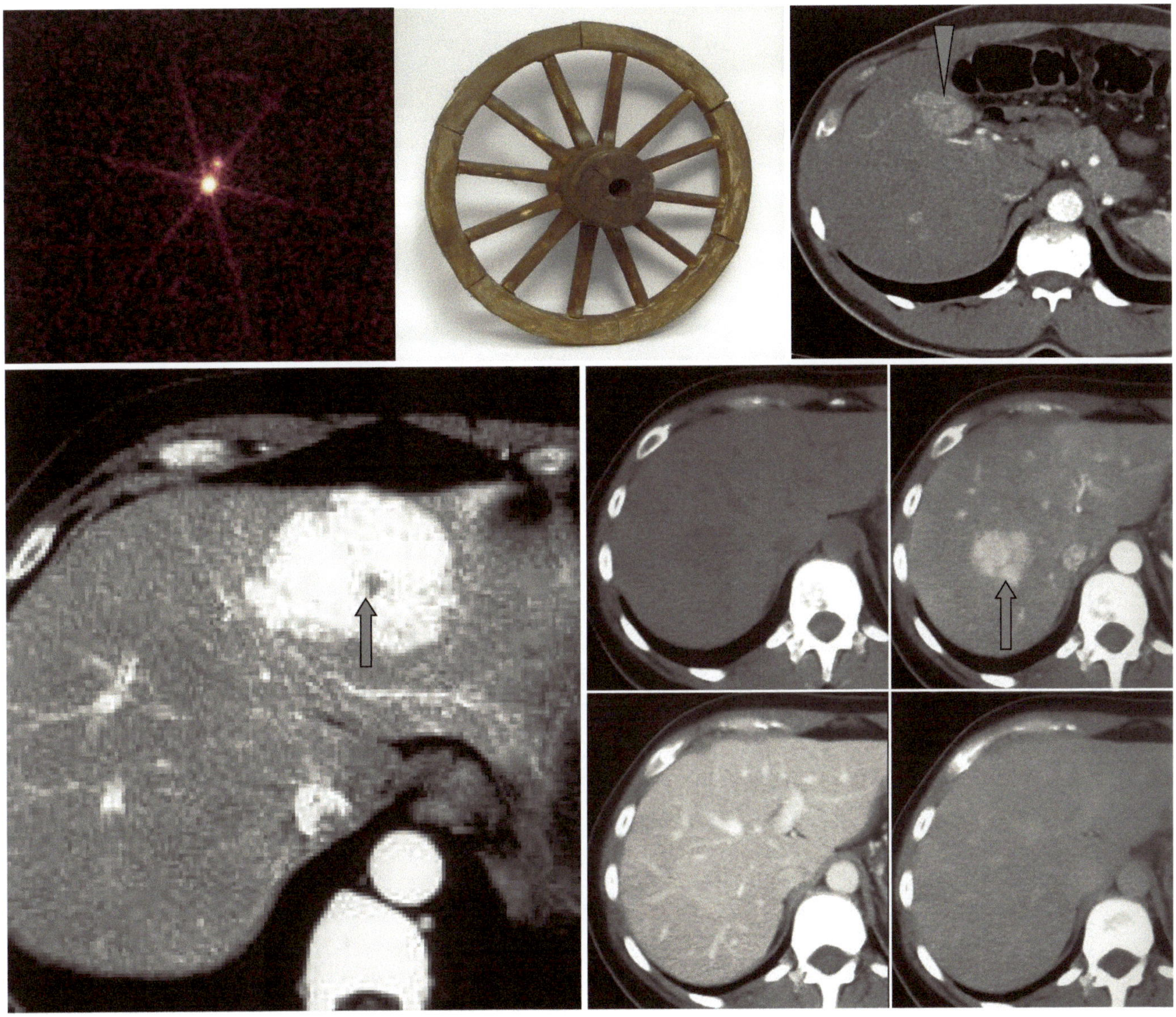

Focal nodular hyperplasia is a benign mass in the liver formed by hyperplastic response to local vascular malformation. Focal nodular hyperplasia is characterized by fast uptake and washout of contrast agent. A typical feature (present in 2/3 of cases) is the central scar depicting a star or the spokes of a wheel, which may enhance in the delayed phase – the "*stellate scar*" sign (↑) or the "*spoke-wheel*" pattern (Δ).

A. Yudin, *Metaphorical Signs in Computed Tomography of Chest and Abdomen*,
DOI 10.1007/978-3-319-04013-4_51,

Funeral Frame Sign, Rim Enhancement, and Target-Like Appearance

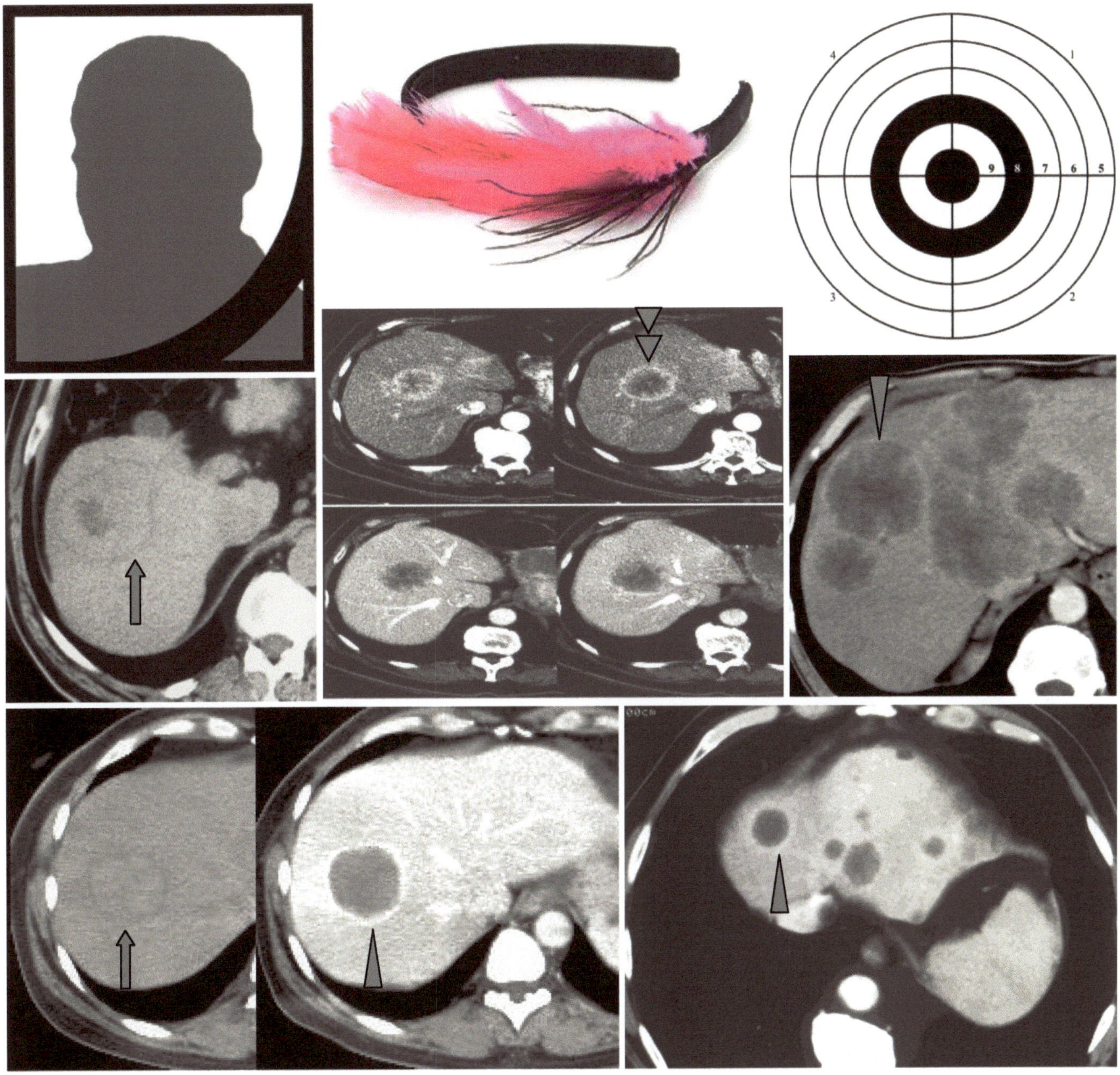

The low-density rim on the periphery of liver masses indicates parenchymal edema around quickly growing tumors, usually metastases, forming the "*funeral frame*" sign (↑) on CT images. After IV enhancement hypovascular metastases may be surrounded by a contrasted rim on the periphery in zones of edema and compression of liver parenchyma – the "*rim enhancement*" (Δ). If the central zone of metastasis is necrotized, the "*target-like appearance*" (►►) may be formed. The "rim enhancement" can also be observed with liver abscesses, especially amebic.

A. Yudin, *Metaphorical Signs in Computed Tomography of Chest and Abdomen*,
DOI 10.1007/978-3-319-04013-4_52, © Springer International Publishing Switzerland 2014

Double Duct Sign

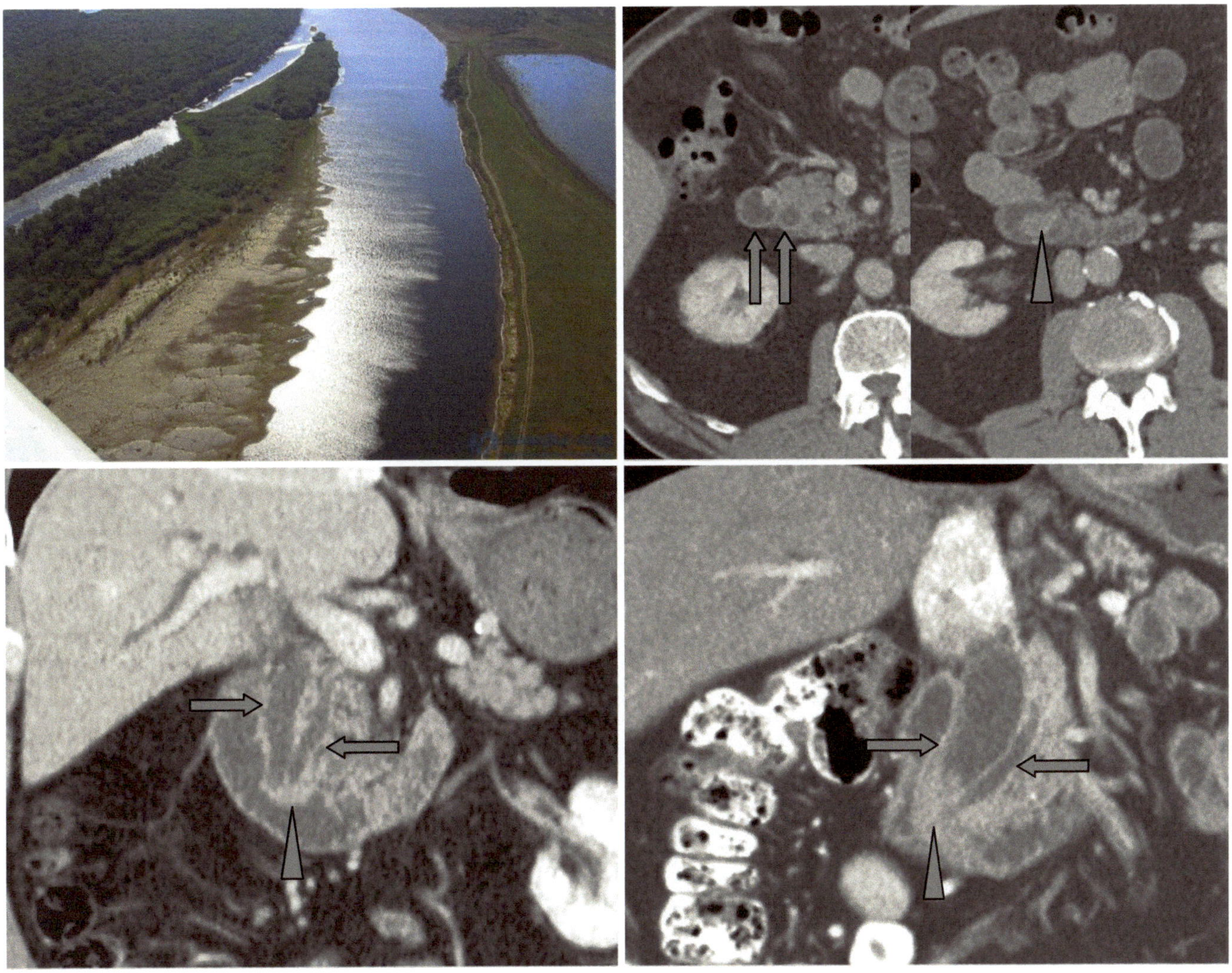

Simultaneous dilation of the common bile duct and the pancreatic duct – the "*double duct*" sign (↑) – is extremely suspicious of an ampullary carcinoma (Δ). The tumor is well defined after oral administration of water and IV enhancement. This sign can also occur in pancreatic head carcinoma invading the ampulla and pancreatitis.

A. Yudin, *Metaphorical Signs in Computed Tomography of Chest and Abdomen*,
DOI 10.1007/978-3-319-04013-4_53, © Springer International Publishing Switzerland 2014

Central Dot Sign

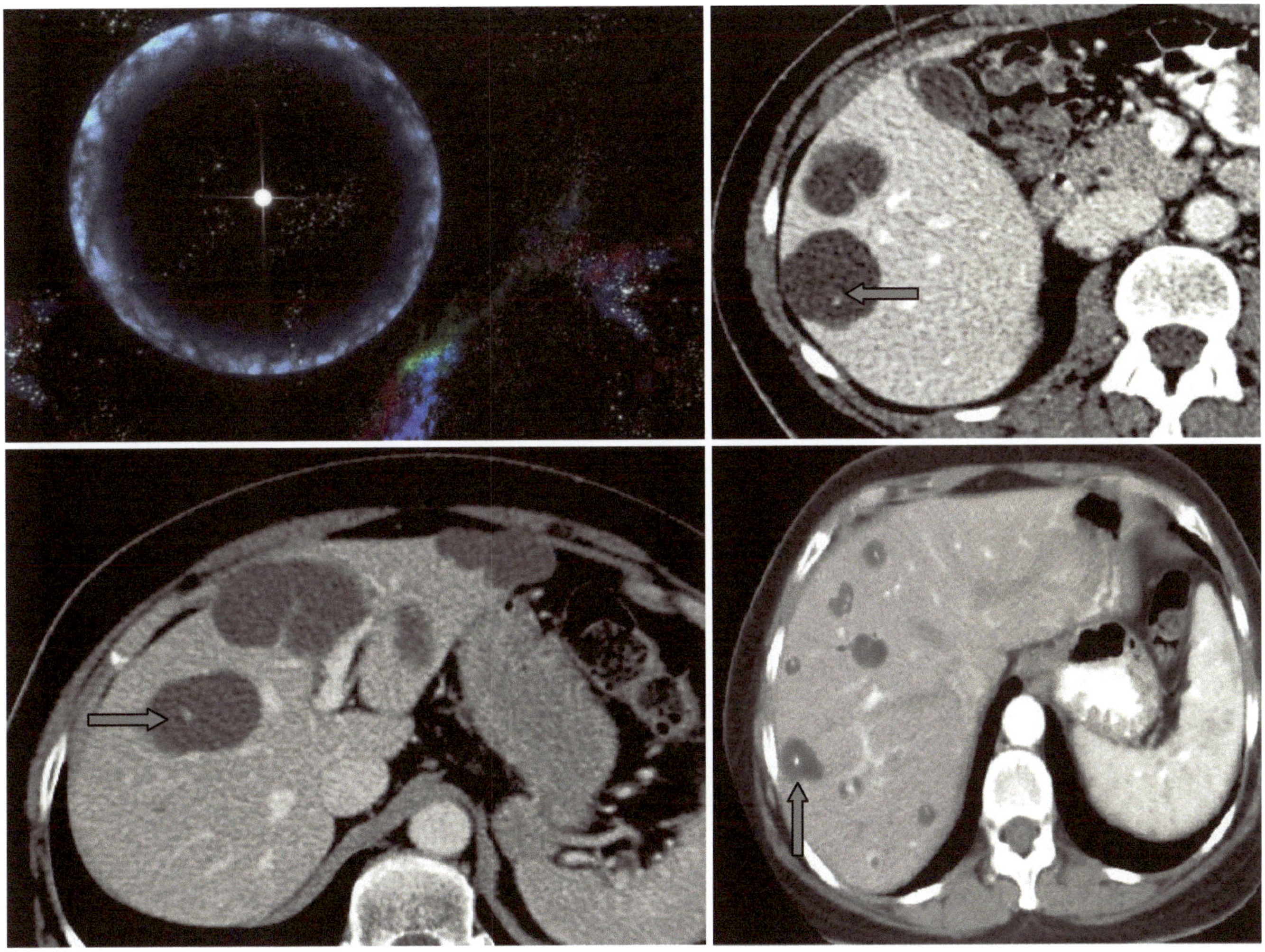

Caroli disease (communicating cavernous biliary ectasia) is the congenital disease characterized by multifocal segmental saccular dilatation of intrahepatic bile ducts. On liver tomograms cystic formations (dilated bile ducts) may be detected with central enhancing dots or stripes (portal vein branches) – the "*central dot*" sign (↑). In some patients hyperdense concrements can be found in dilated bile ducts. The similar picture can be seen in mycotic liver affection.

A. Yudin, *Metaphorical Signs in Computed Tomography of Chest and Abdomen*,
DOI 10.1007/978-3-319-04013-4_54, © Springer International Publishing Switzerland 2014

Mercedes-Benz Sign

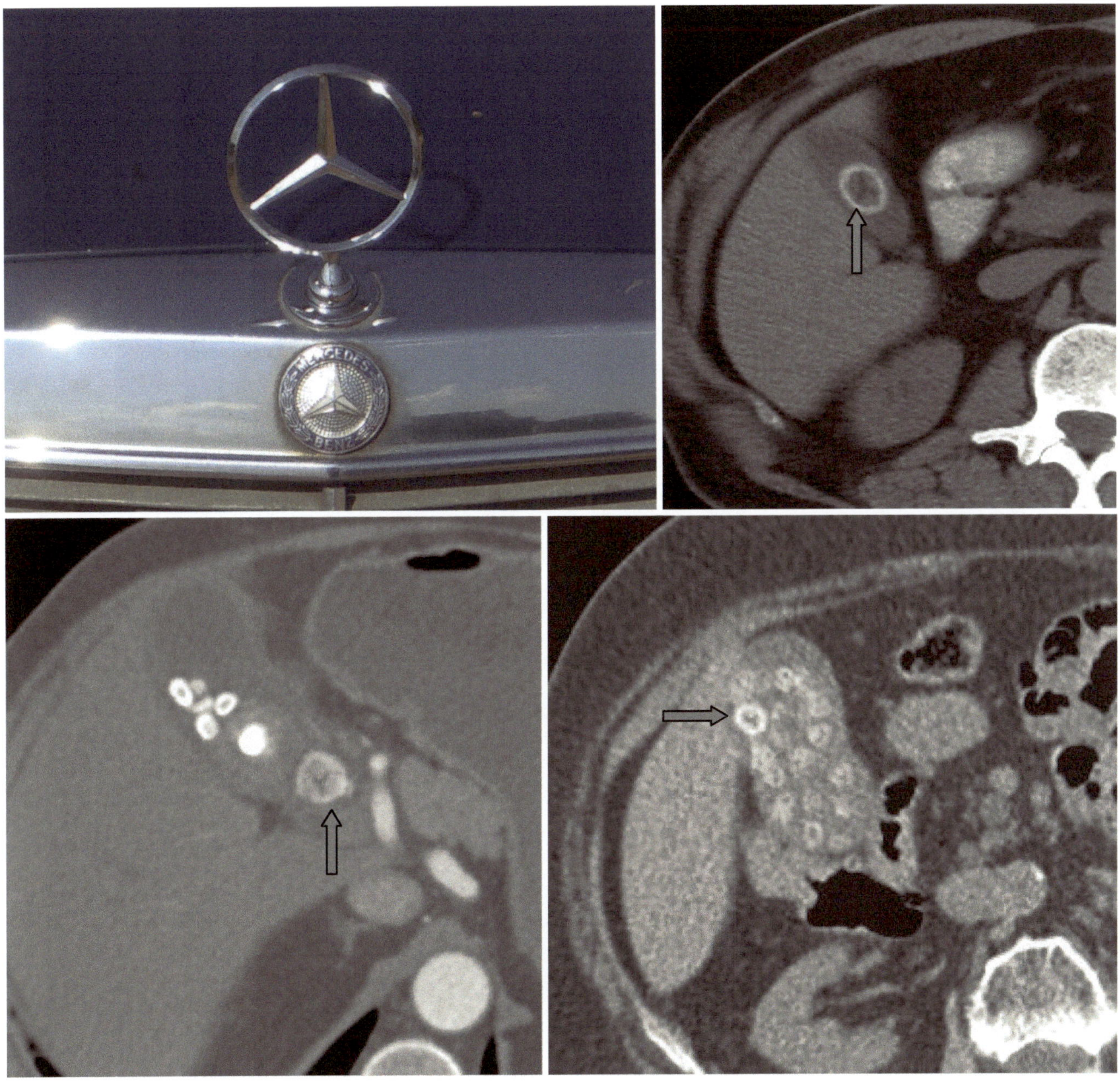

Some gallbladder stones contain gas in the central zone and frequently have the form of a three-beam star – the "*Mercedes-Benz*" sign (↑). There is an assumption that during the evolution the central part of concrements reduces more significantly than the peripheral. Thus, cracks may be formed and filled with gas because of a vacuum phenomenon. Anyhow, this sign has no urgent potential.

A. Yudin, *Metaphorical Signs in Computed Tomography of Chest and Abdomen*,
DOI 10.1007/978-3-319-04013-4_55, © Springer International Publishing Switzerland 2014

Porcelain or Incrusted Gallbladder Sign

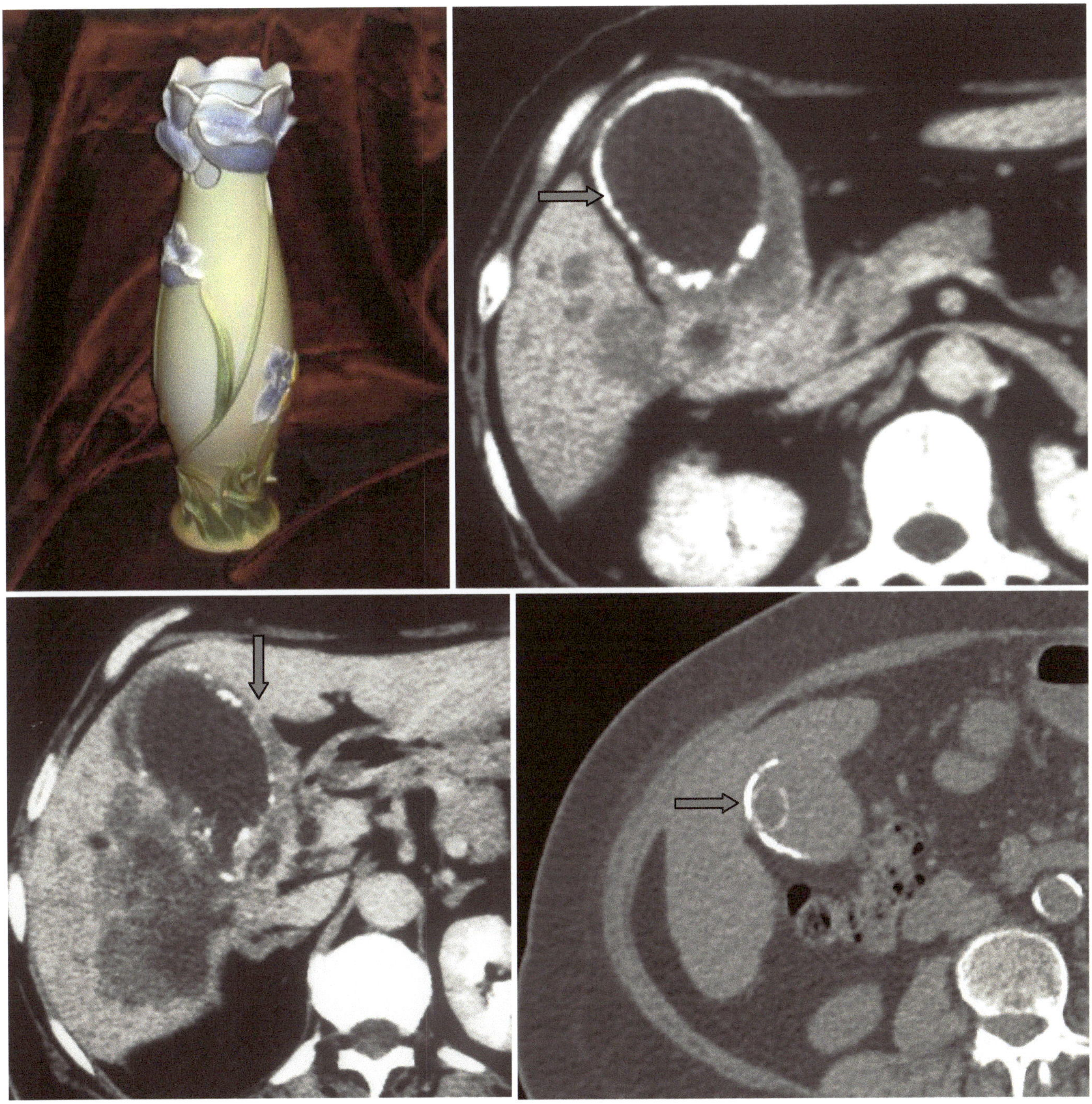

It is considered that the curvilinear calcification in the gallbladder wall – the "*porcelain gallbladder*" sign or the "*incrusted gallbladder*" sign (↑) – is a sign of chronic cholecystitis. However, during CT the majority of such patients demonstrate gallbladder carcinoma with soft tissue mass frequently involving liver parenchyma.

A. Yudin, *Metaphorical Signs in Computed Tomography of Chest and Abdomen*,
DOI 10.1007/978-3-319-04013-4_56, © Springer International Publishing Switzerland 2014

Annular Pancreas

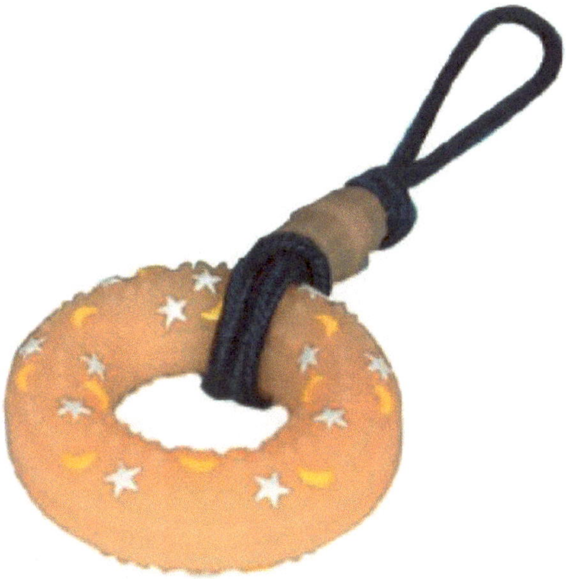

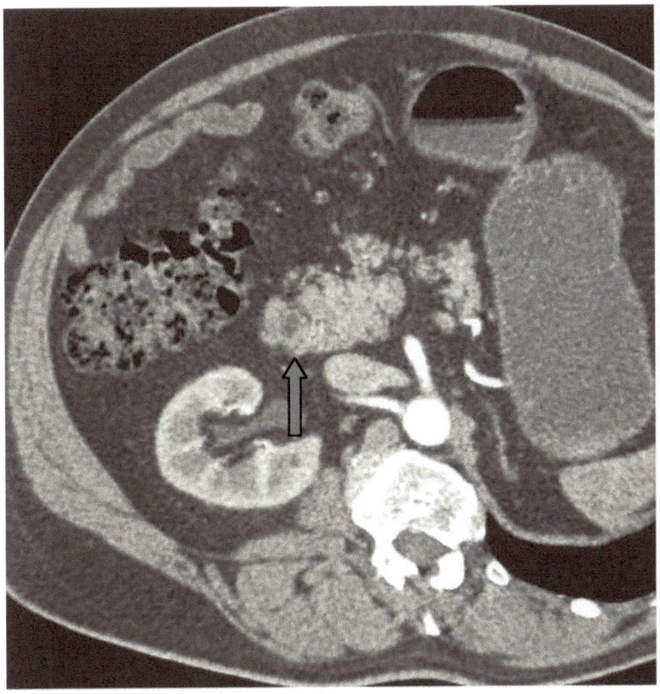

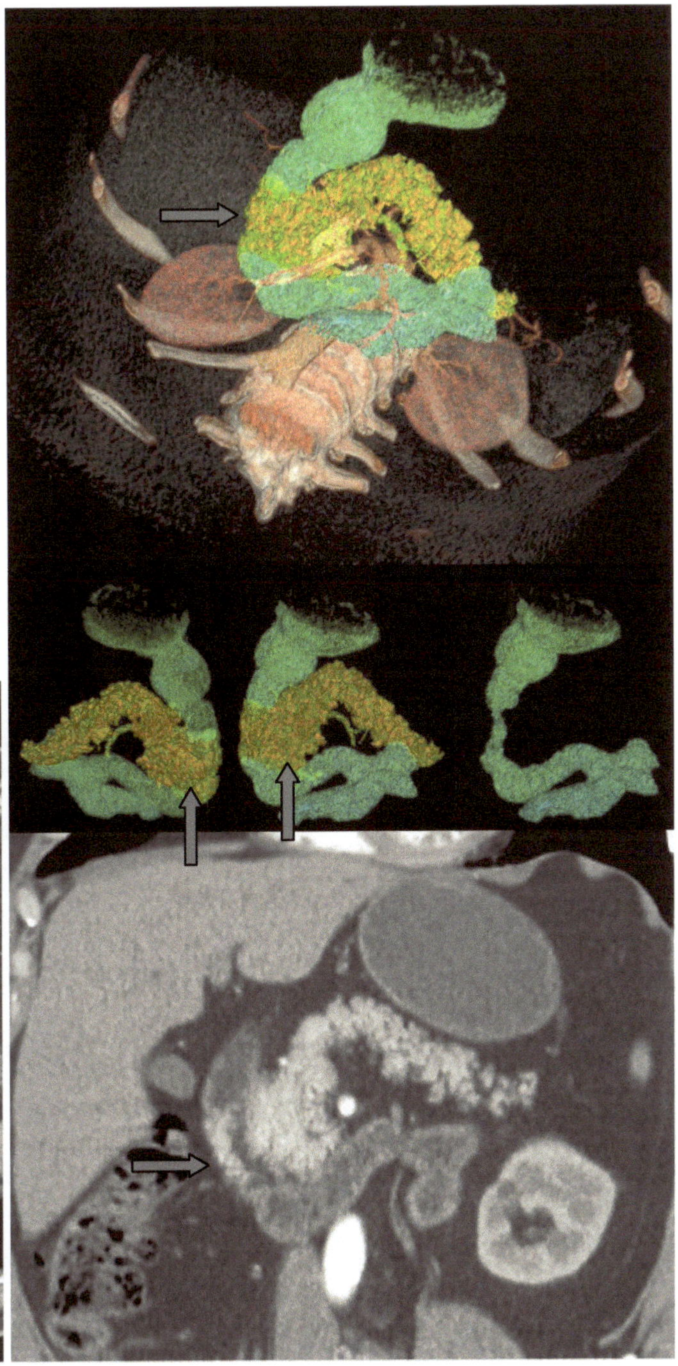

Annular pancreas is a variant of development. The normal tissue of the pancreatic head and common bile duct envelop the descending part of the duodenum (↑). If detected in childhood, it may be combined with some developmental anomalies in 75 % of cases. In adult age such complications as pancreatitis and gastric and duodenal ulcers may occur.

A. Yudin, *Metaphorical Signs in Computed Tomography of Chest and Abdomen*,
DOI 10.1007/978-3-319-04013-4_57,

Lake Chain Sign or String of Beads Sign and Pancreas with Sausage-Like Form and Hypodense Halo

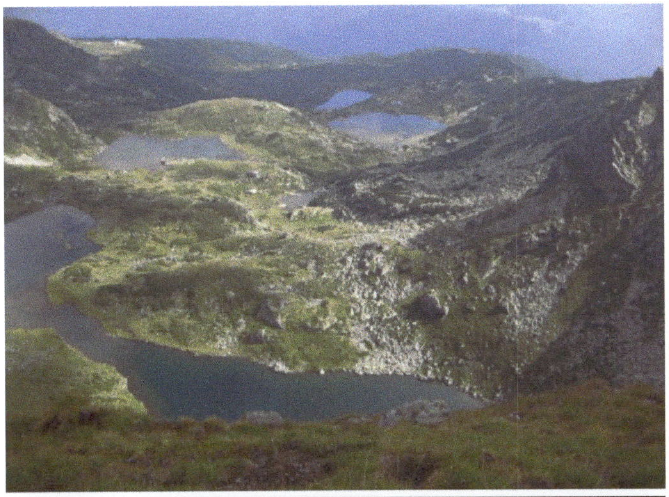

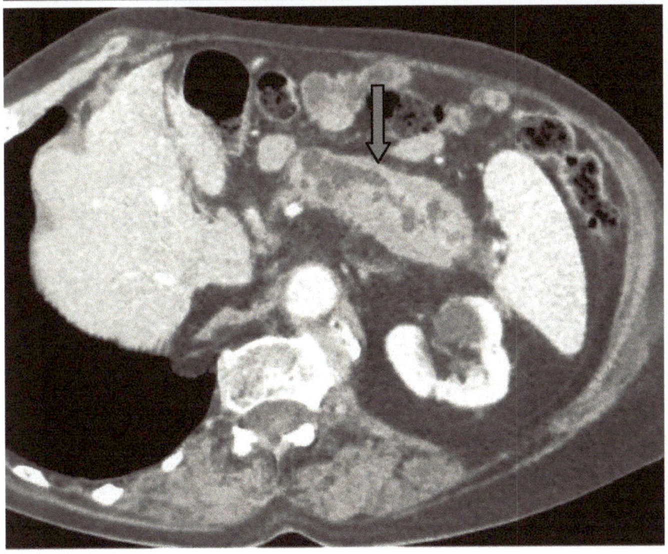

In chronic pancreatitis duct dilatation is present in 50 % of patients because of atrophic parenchymal changes. The lumen is often dilated irregularly as a result of cicatricial deformity forming the "*lake chain*" sign (↑) or the "*string of beads*" sign.

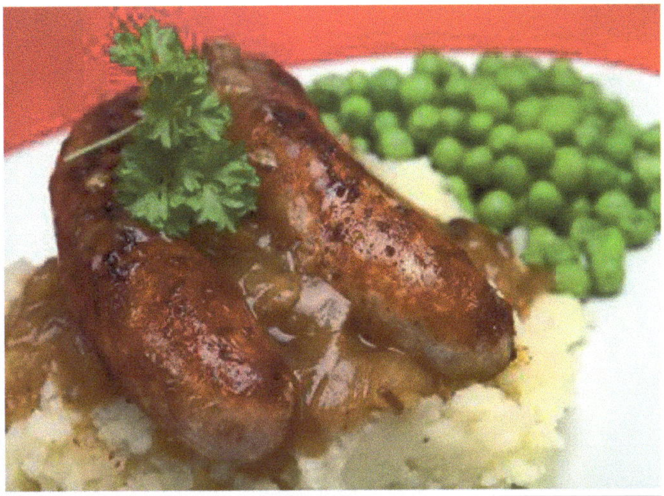

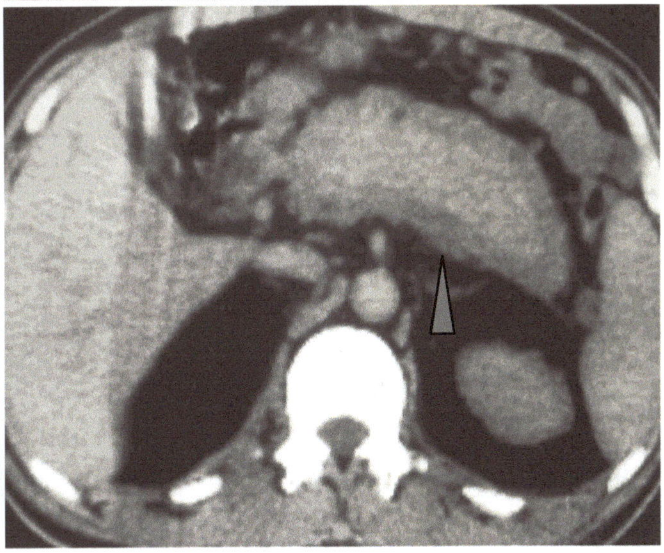

In autoimmune pancreatitis, the duct is narrowed and not defined, but the gland is enlarged, loses its natural lobulation, and acquires a *sausage-like form* with *a hypodense halo* (Δ) on the periphery. Autoimmune pancreatitis has a good response to corticosteroid treatment.

A. Yudin, *Metaphorical Signs in Computed Tomography of Chest and Abdomen*,
DOI 10.1007/978-3-319-04013-4_58, © Springer International Publishing Switzerland 2014

Honeycomb or Spongelike Mass and Spoke-Wheel Sign

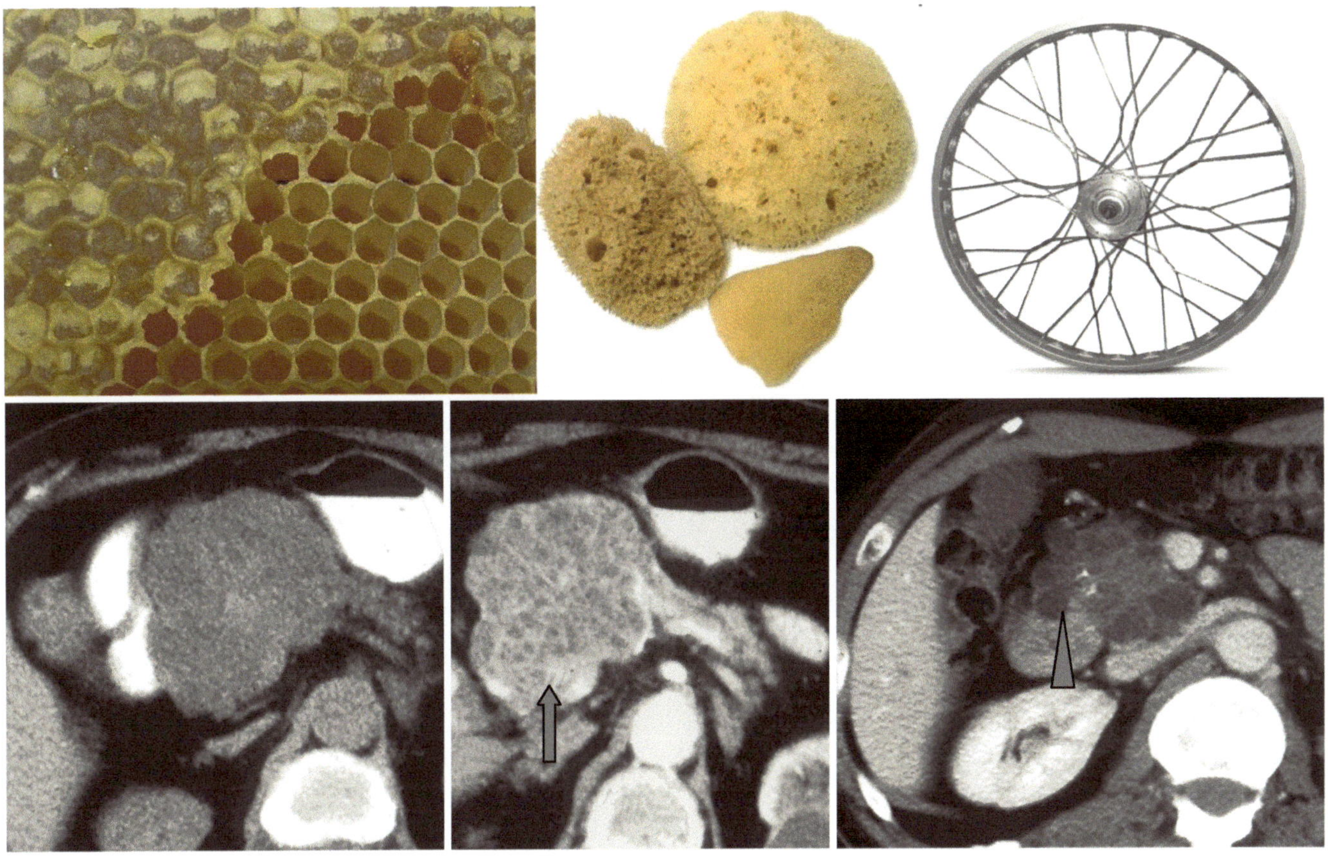

Pancreatic serous cystadenoma (serous microcystic adenoma) is a benign tumor which consists of a considerable amount of small cysts (more than 6 and less than 2 cm in diameter), more common in the pancreatic head. After IV enhancement the septa emphasize the contours of fine cysts forming *honeycomb* or *spongelike mass* (↑) but sometimes can prevail over cysts, creating a view of a solid mass. Central soft tissue scar, frequently with calcification, is seldom found. The septa spreading from it always form the "*spoke-wheel*" sign (Δ).

A. Yudin, *Metaphorical Signs in Computed Tomography of Chest and Abdomen*,
DOI 10.1007/978-3-319-04013-4_59, © Springer International Publishing Switzerland 2014

Fetal Lobulation or Lobation and Column of Bertin Hypertrophy

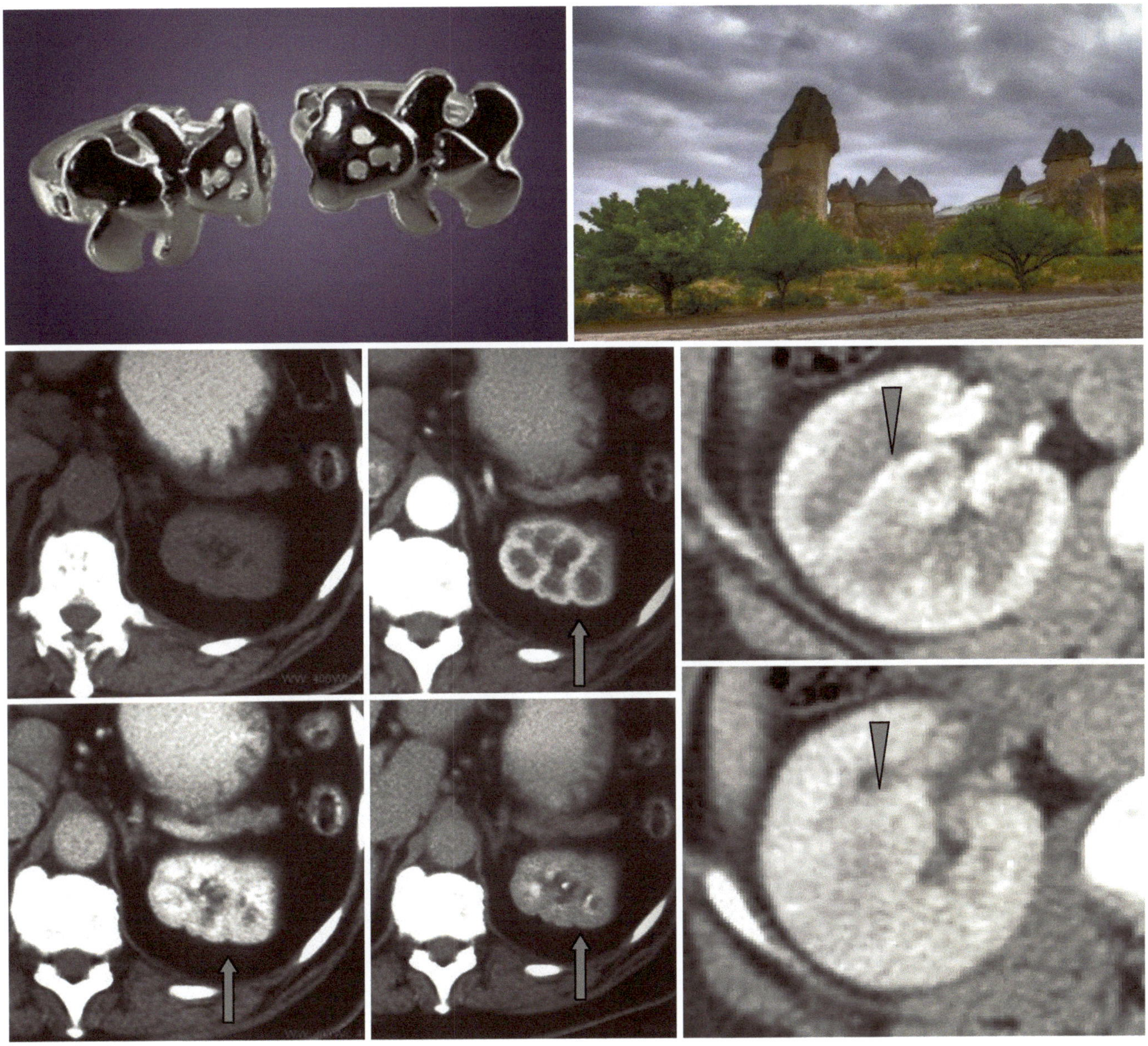

Fetal and early-age children kidneys consist of separate lobes delimited by deep sulci from each other – the so-called *"fetal lobulation or lobation"* (↑). The kidneys have humpy surfaces. As children grow, the lobes coalesce forming a smooth surface of kidneys in adults, but in 4–5 % of patients, the fetal lobulation remains. During CT normal enhancement of the cortical zone must be observed but with deep surface clefts in projections of Bertin septa.

Column of Bertin (Δ) represents a hypertrophied wide and long cortical band deeply penetrating between the pyramids of medullary tissue.

Both developmental variants have no clinical value, but they are often mistaken for renal tumors.

A. Yudin, *Metaphorical Signs in Computed Tomography of Chest and Abdomen*,
DOI 10.1007/978-3-319-04013-4_60, © Springer International Publishing Switzerland 2014

Horseshoe Kidney

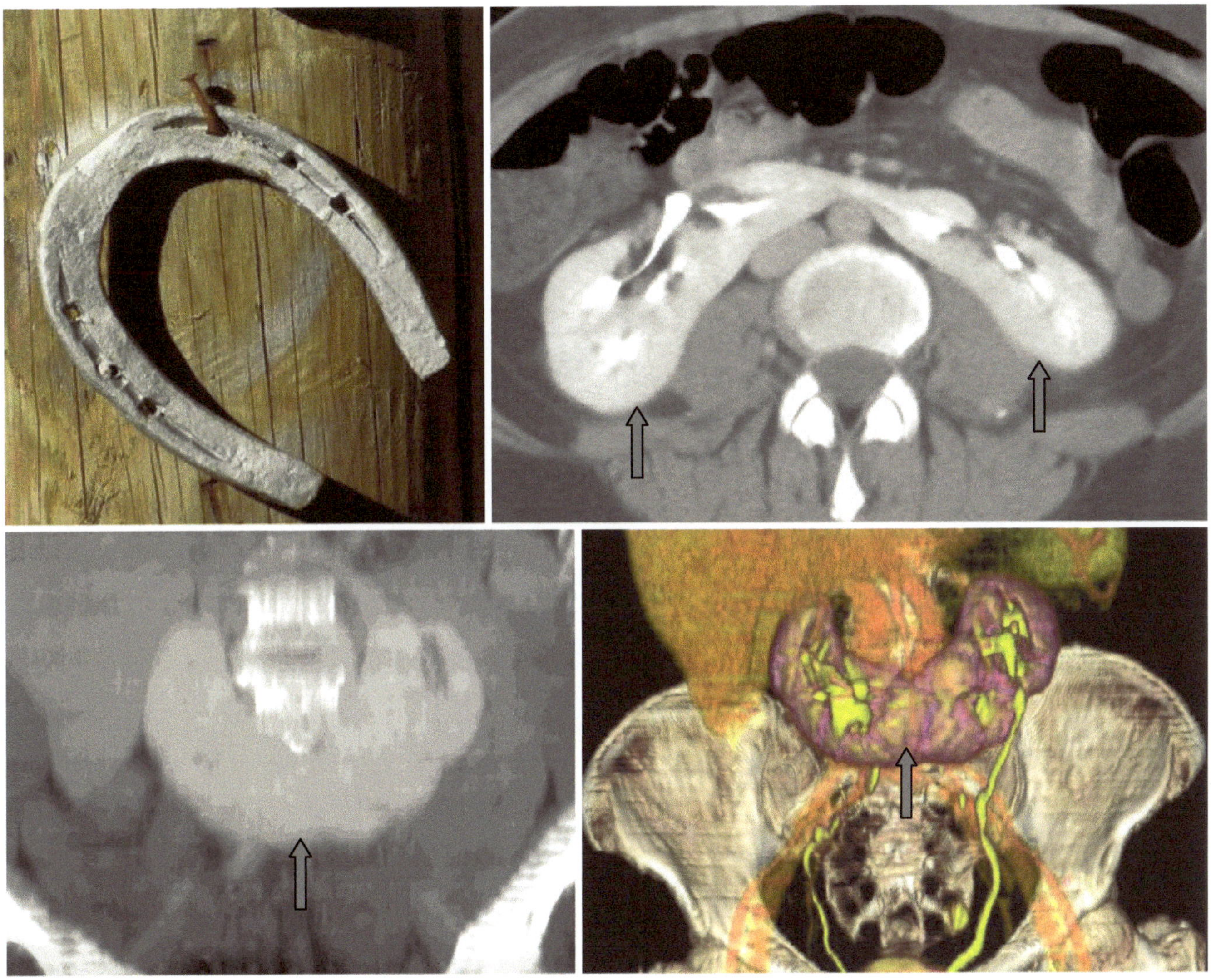

The *horseshoe kidney* (↑) is a congenital anomaly, at which kidneys are united by the isthmus in the region of lower poles. There are two variants of coalescence: median or symmetrical (most common) and lateral or asymmetrical. This condition is associated with high probability of traumatic damage, development of Wilms tumors, renal cell carcinomas, vesicoureteral reflux, and urolithiasis.

A. Yudin, *Metaphorical Signs in Computed Tomography of Chest and Abdomen*,
DOI 10.1007/978-3-319-04013-4_61, © Springer International Publishing Switzerland 2014

White Pyramids Sign

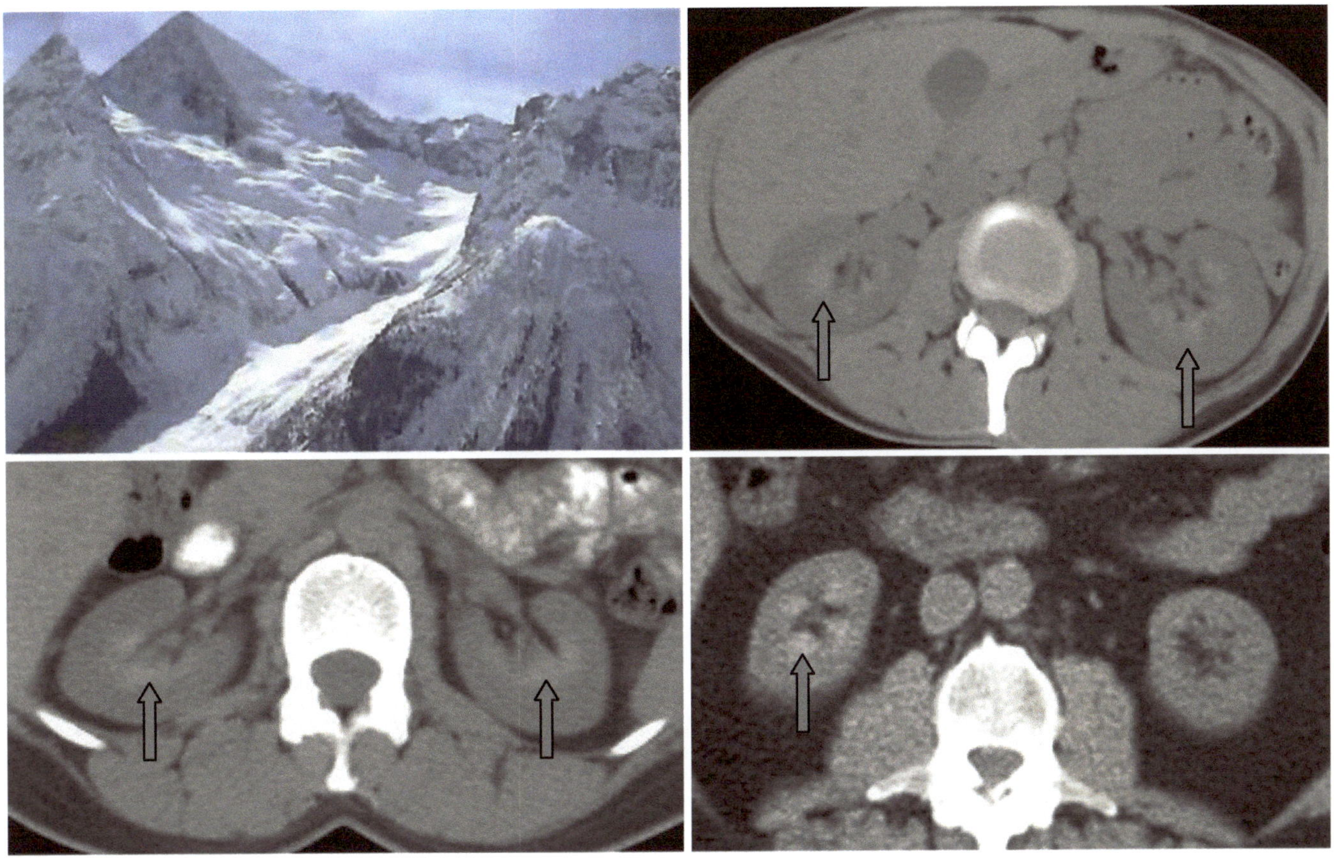

Quite often on native images renal pyramids look hyperdense in comparison with other tissues – the "*white pyramids*" sign (↑) – which most likely depicts concentrated urine. The presence of this sign only in one kidney may serve as an additional indirect indicator of obstructive uropathy in the opposite kidney (possible manifestation of tubular hydronephrosis).

A. Yudin, *Metaphorical Signs in Computed Tomography of Chest and Abdomen*,
DOI 10.1007/978-3-319-04013-4_62,

Claw Sign or Beak Sign

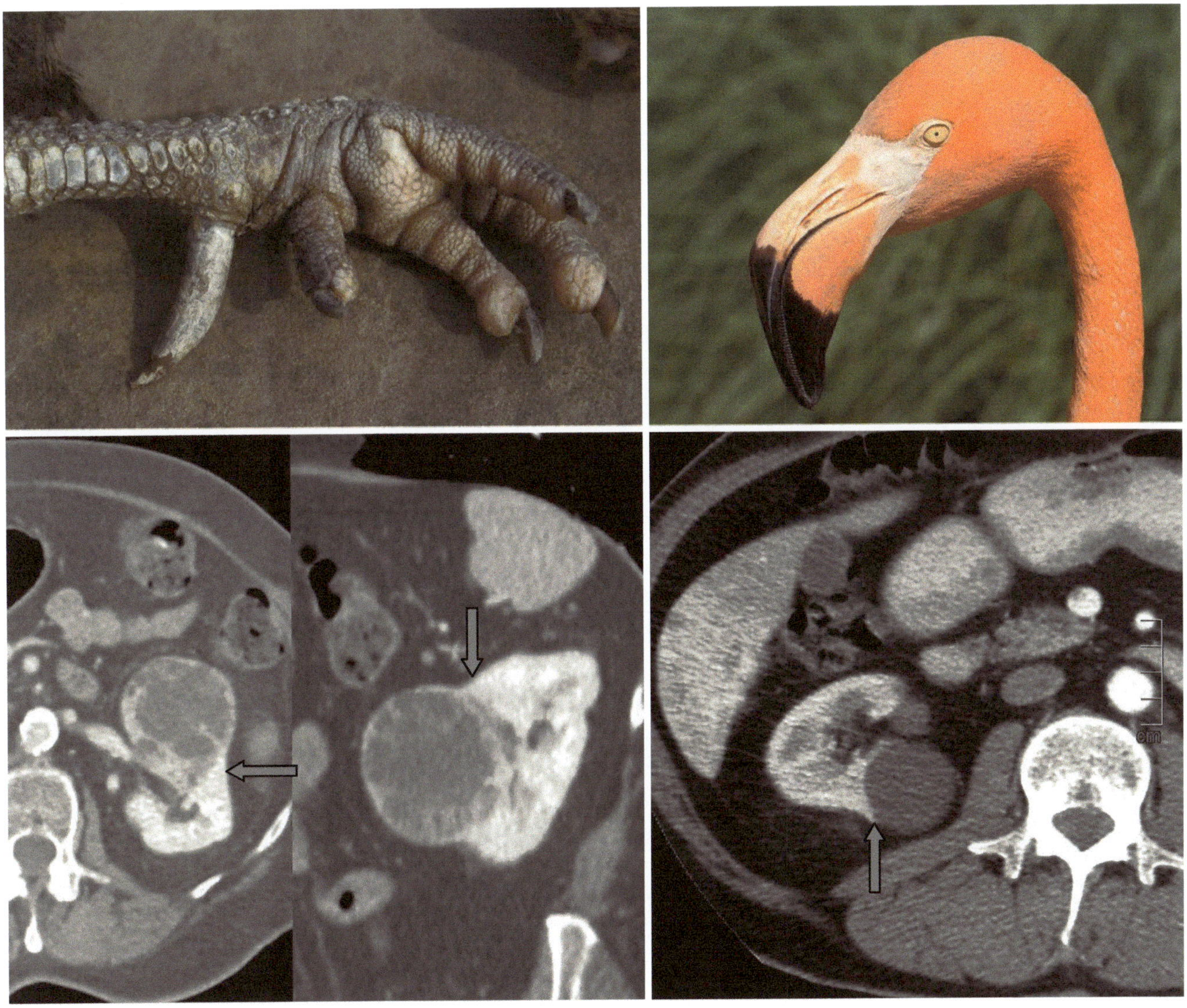

In cases when some masses or cysts grow and bulge from renal parenchyma, the normal tissue covers their contours with the formation of acute angles – the "*claw*" sign or the "*beak*" sign (↑). If the formation is nonorganic but adjoins the organ and probably compresses it, the organ contour will be wrapped inside. This sign does not indicate the benign origin of the lesion but shows the expansive variant of growth.

A. Yudin, *Metaphorical Signs in Computed Tomography of Chest and Abdomen*,
DOI 10.1007/978-3-319-04013-4_63, © Springer International Publishing Switzerland 2014

Faceless Kidney Sign

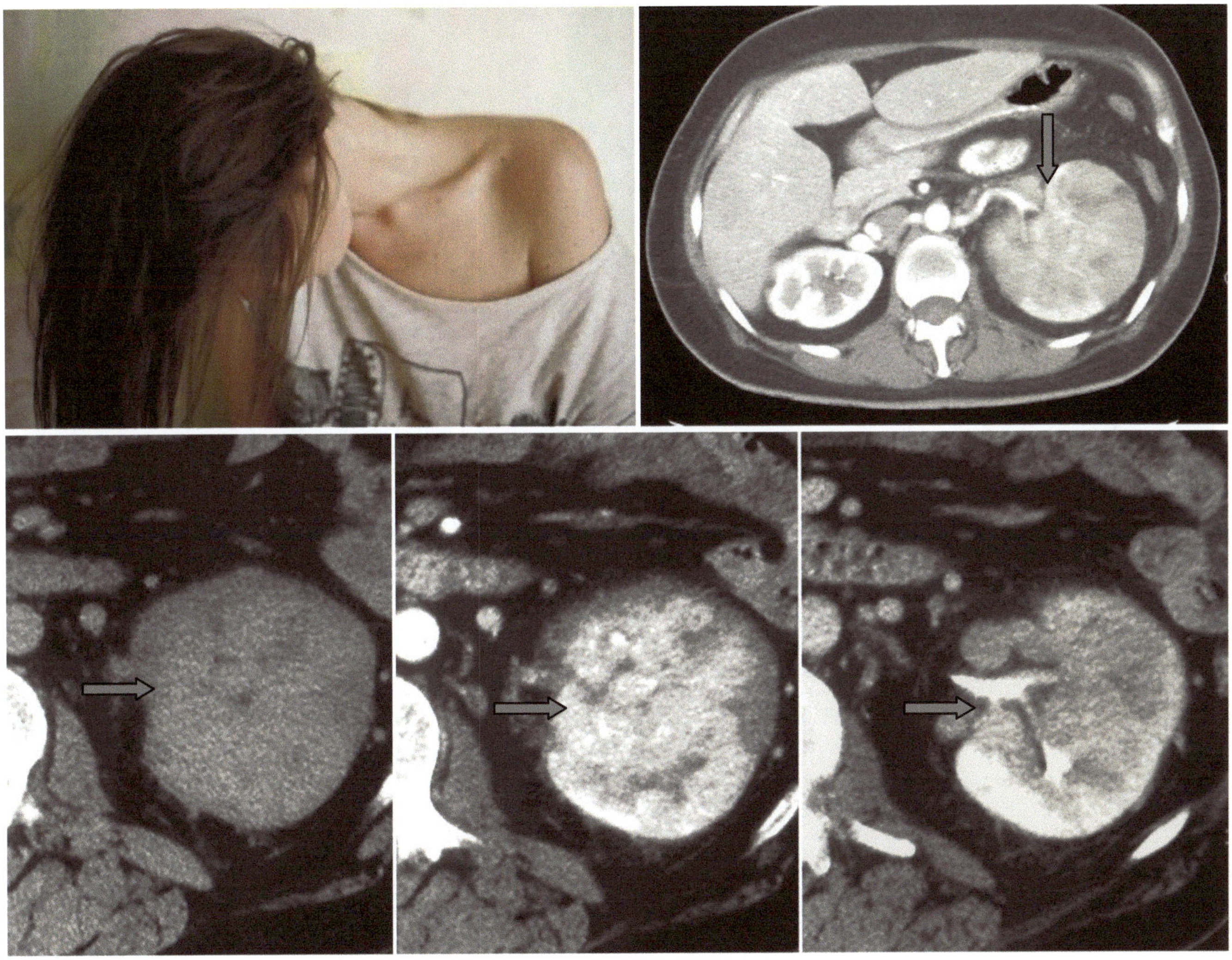

Loss of differentiation of the renal pelvis because of any obliterative process leads to formation of the "*faceless kidney*" sign (↑). First, this sign was described in patients with incomplete kidney duplication. Most frequent causes of obliteration of pelvic fatty tissue are lymphomas and transitional cell carcinomas.

A. Yudin, *Metaphorical Signs in Computed Tomography of Chest and Abdomen*,
DOI 10.1007/978-3-319-04013-4_64, © Springer International Publishing Switzerland 2014

Swiss Cheese Sign

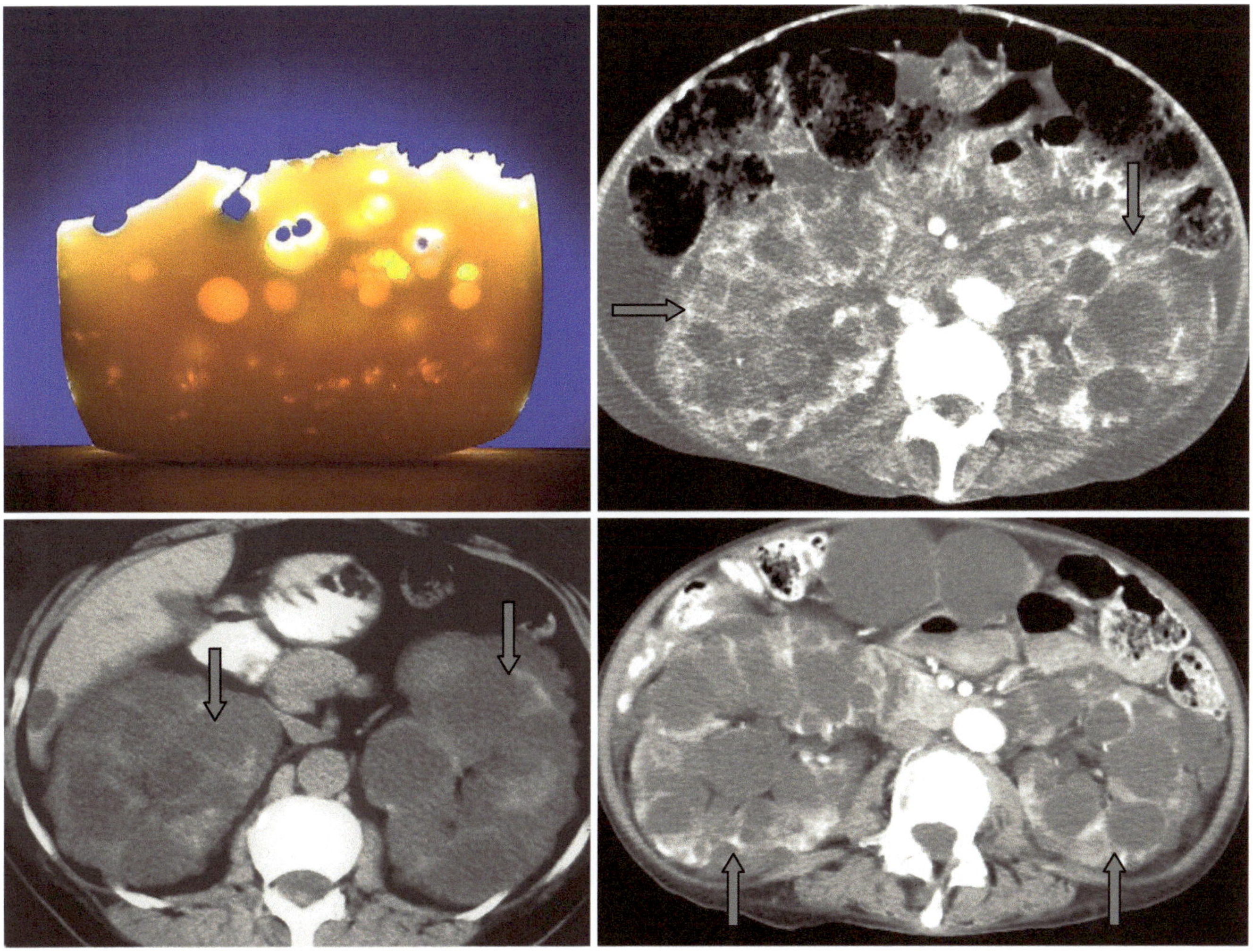

Considerably enlarged kidneys with innumerable cysts of different sizes, some of them demonstrate hemorrhages and wall calcifications, form the "*Swiss cheese*" sign (↑) which is a typical manifestation of autosomal dominant polycystic kidneys disease. Without adequate treatment by 40–50 years of age, patients develop renal failure because of the replacement of parenchyma by cysts. Multisystem manifestations may also involve the liver, pancreas, spleen, ovaries, and testes.

A. Yudin, *Metaphorical Signs in Computed Tomography of Chest and Abdomen*,
DOI 10.1007/978-3-319-04013-4_65, © Springer International Publishing Switzerland 2014

Stellate Scar Sign or Starlike Scar Sign and Spoke-Wheel Pattern

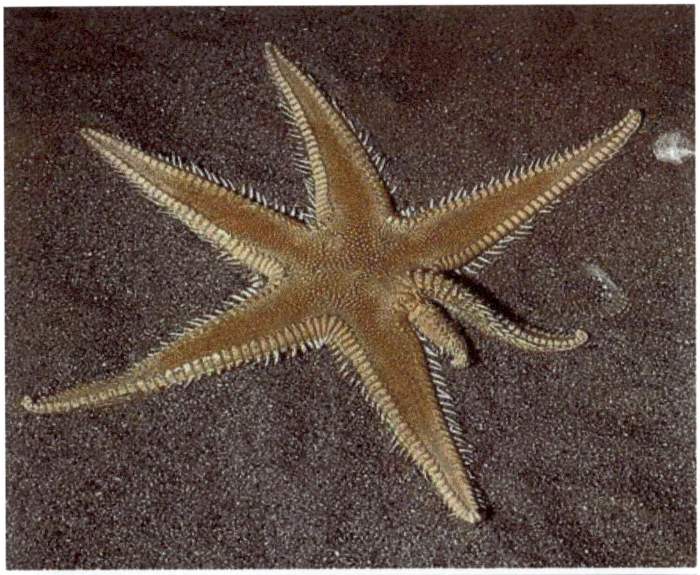
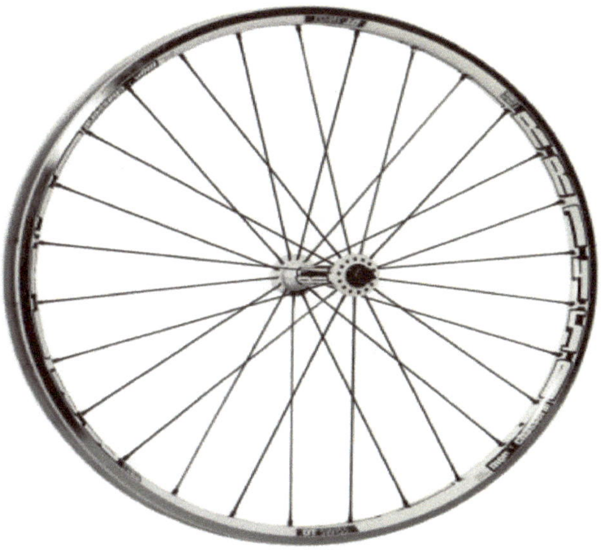
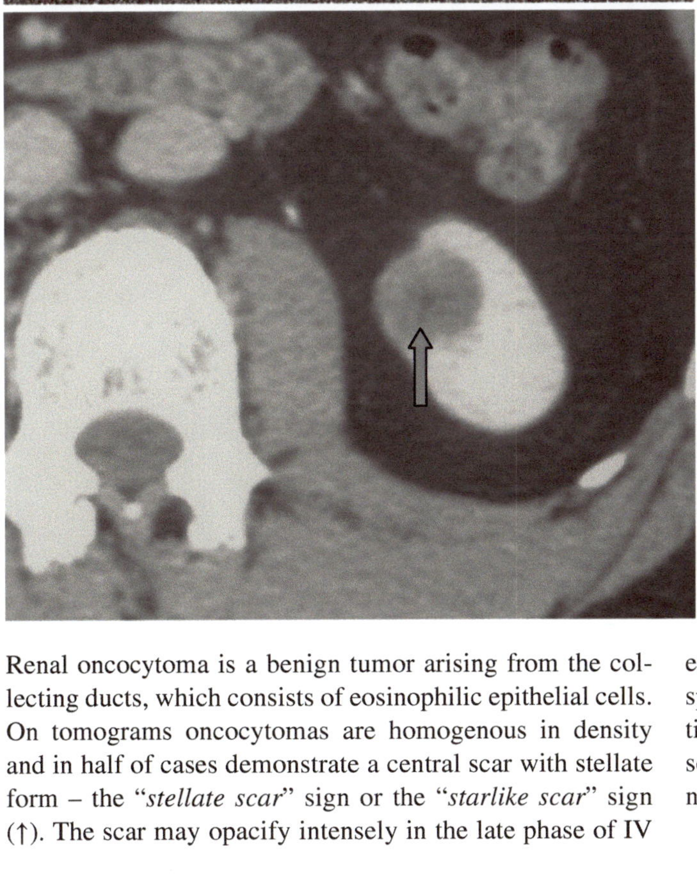
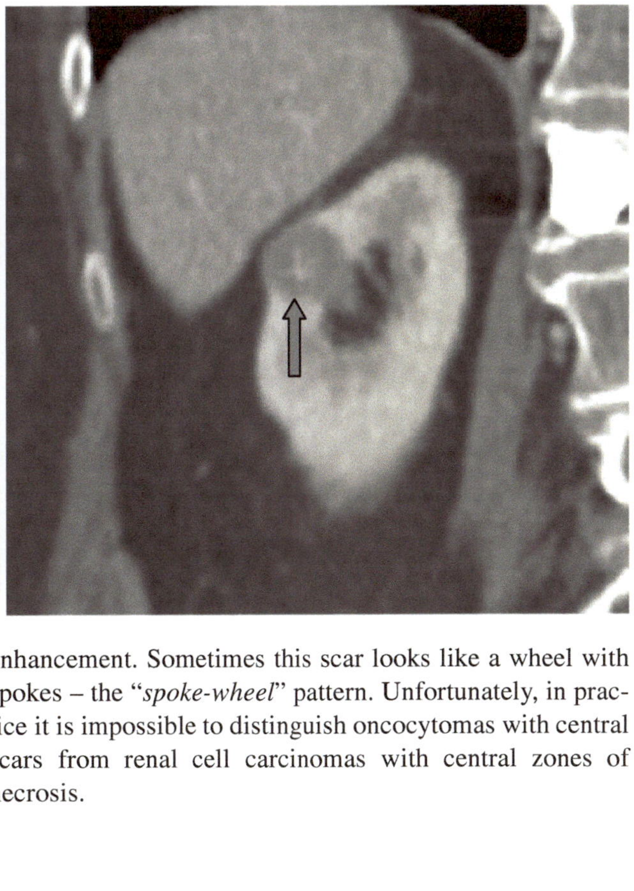

Renal oncocytoma is a benign tumor arising from the collecting ducts, which consists of eosinophilic epithelial cells. On tomograms oncocytomas are homogenous in density and in half of cases demonstrate a central scar with stellate form – the "*stellate scar*" sign or the "*starlike scar*" sign (↑). The scar may opacify intensely in the late phase of IV enhancement. Sometimes this scar looks like a wheel with spokes – the "*spoke-wheel*" pattern. Unfortunately, in practice it is impossible to distinguish oncocytomas with central scars from renal cell carcinomas with central zones of necrosis.

A. Yudin, *Metaphorical Signs in Computed Tomography of Chest and Abdomen*,
DOI 10.1007/978-3-319-04013-4_66, © Springer International Publishing Switzerland 2014

Fan Sign, Wedge-Shaped or Striated Enhancement, and Patchy Nephrogram

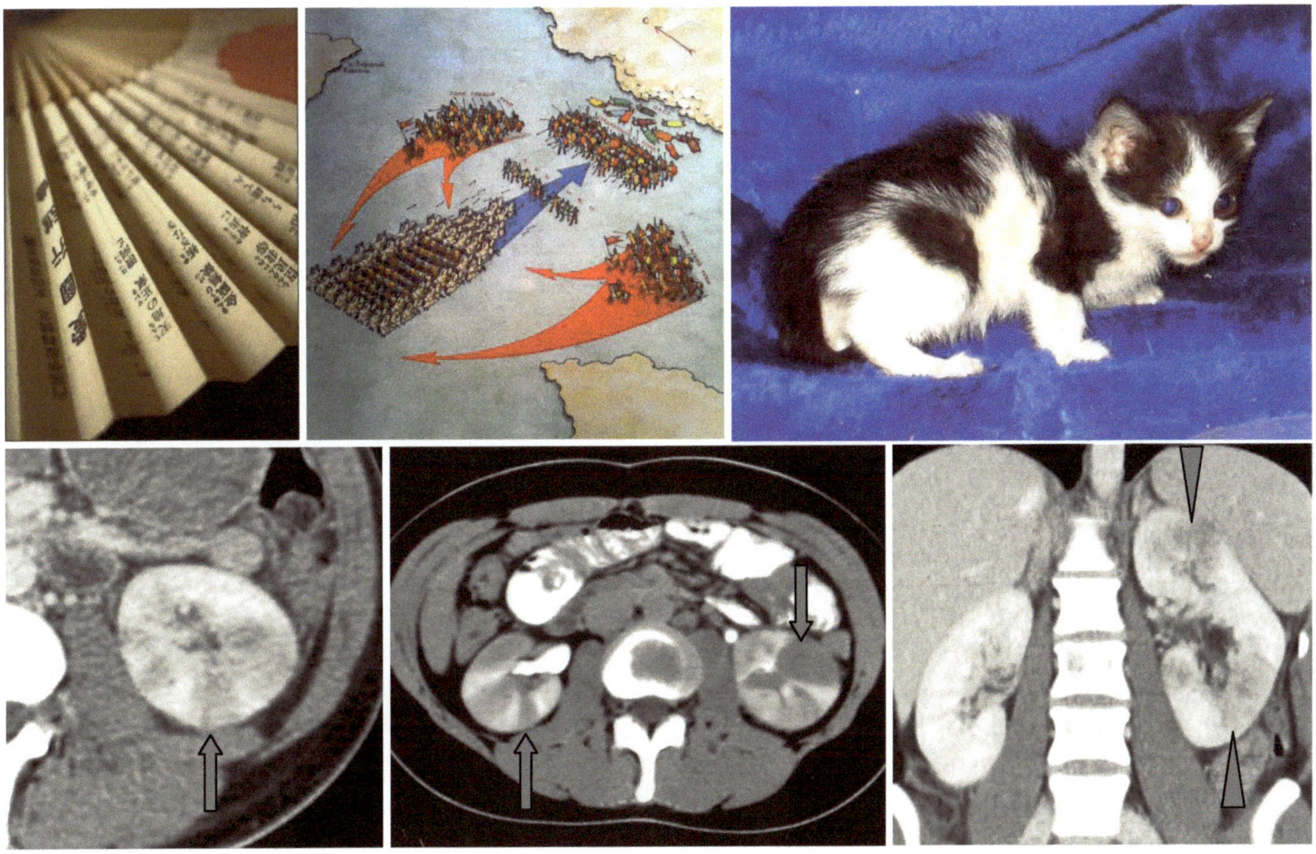

In acute pyelonephritis in the parenchymal phase of IV enhancement, fan- or wedge-like, striated, or patchy zones of low attenuation may be found forming the "*fan*" sign (↑), "*wedge-shaped* or *striated* enhancement", or "*patchy nephrogram*" (Δ). These areas correspond to necrosis and edema. In the delayed phase of enhancement, the zones of previously low density can slightly enhance. Similar changes in the kidneys occur in embolism, vasculitis, atherosclerosis, and trauma. Thus, clinical correlation is necessary for differentiation of these pathologic conditions.

A. Yudin, *Metaphorical Signs in Computed Tomography of Chest and Abdomen*,
DOI 10.1007/978-3-319-04013-4_67, © Springer International Publishing Switzerland 2014

Medullary Sponge Kidney and Paintbrush Appearance

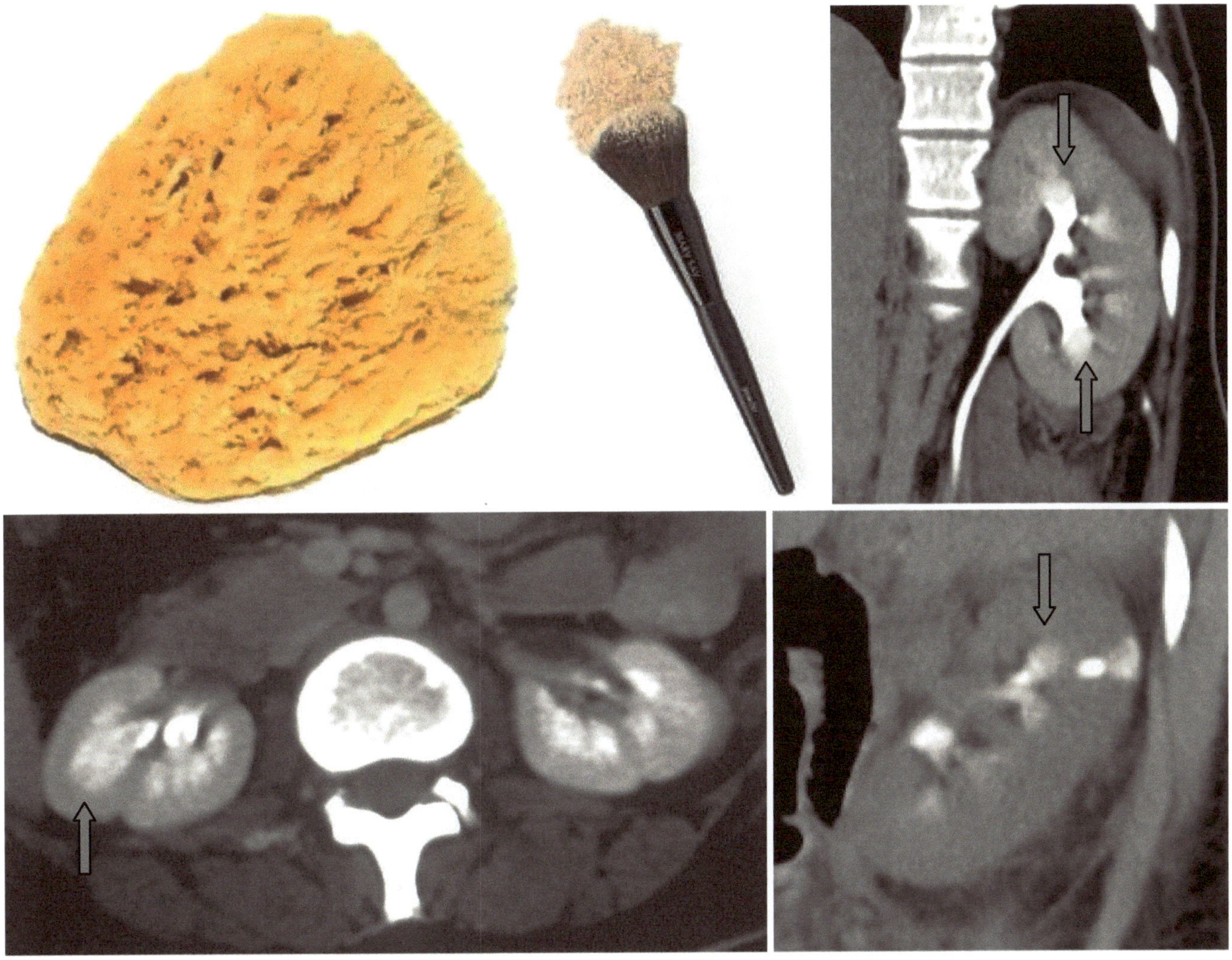

The "*medullary sponge kidney*" or renal tubular ectasia is a degenerative transformation consisting in cystic dilation of collecting ducts in the renal medulla. On tomograms in the excretory phase of enhancement, the delay of contrast agent in widened pyramid tubules is seen forming a "*paintbrush appearance*" (↑). This condition can be complicated by medullary nephrocalcinosis, urolithiasis, and abscesses. The changes are most clearly seen with thin collimation of X-rays and multiplanar reconstructions.

A. Yudin, *Metaphorical Signs in Computed Tomography of Chest and Abdomen*,
DOI 10.1007/978-3-319-04013-4_68, © Springer International Publishing Switzerland 2014

Putty Kidney Sign

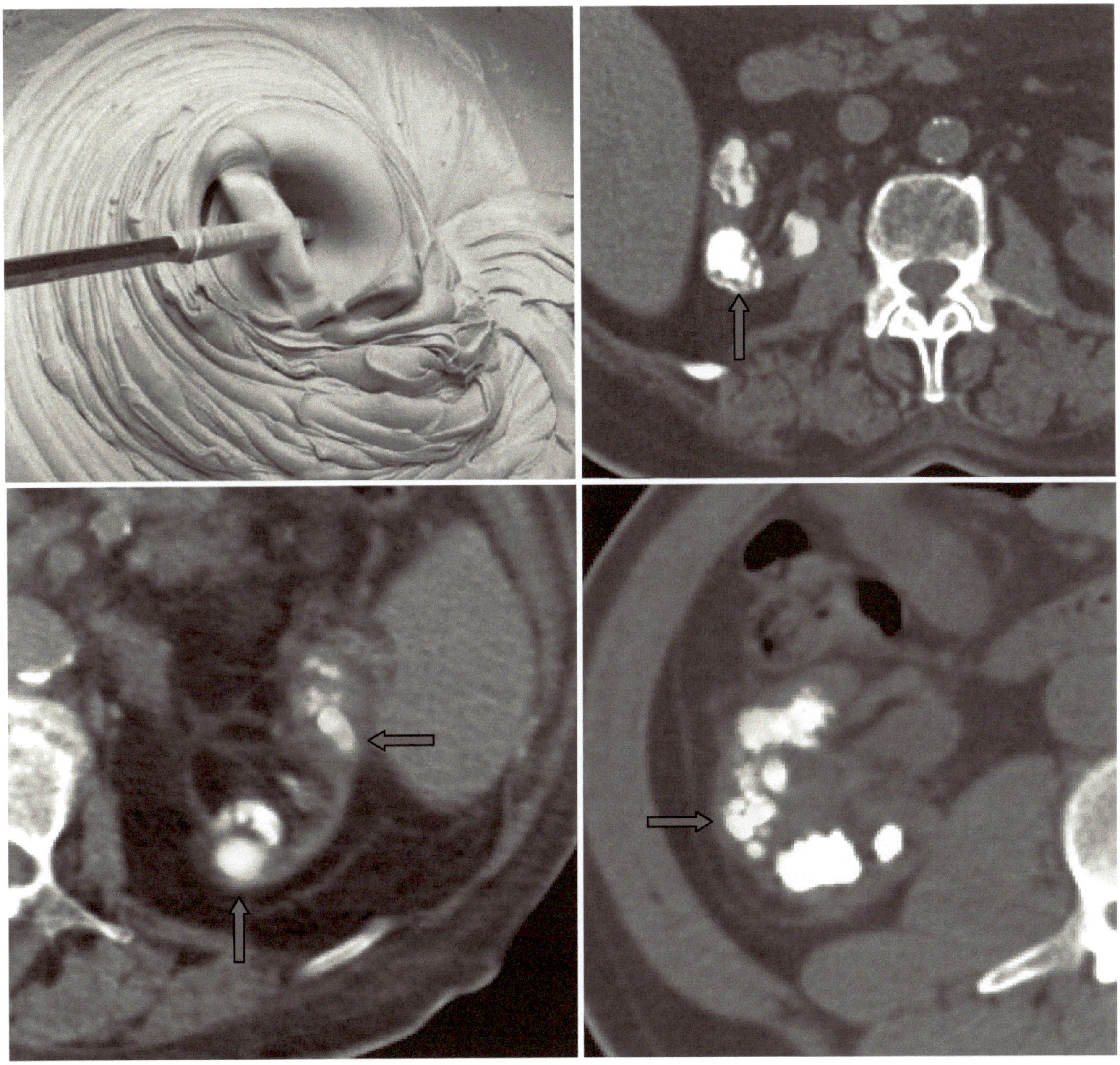

"*Putty kidney*" is pronounced calcification (↑) of nonfunctioning kidney parenchyma (autonephrectomy), caused by end-stage tuberculosis.

A. Yudin, *Metaphorical Signs in Computed Tomography of Chest and Abdomen*,
DOI 10.1007/978-3-319-04013-4_69,

Cortical Rim Sign and Reversed Rim Sign

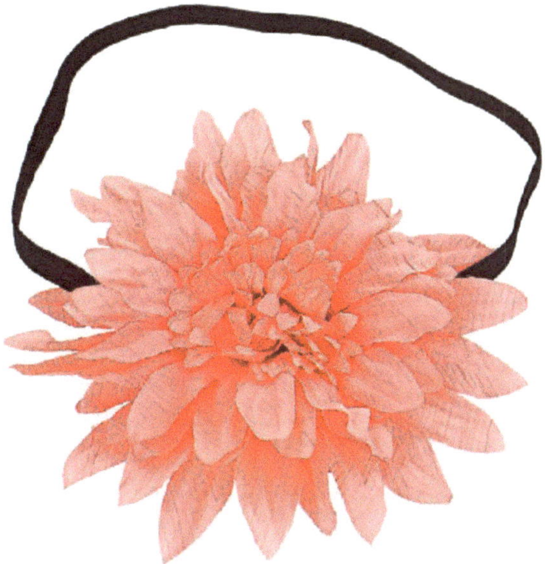

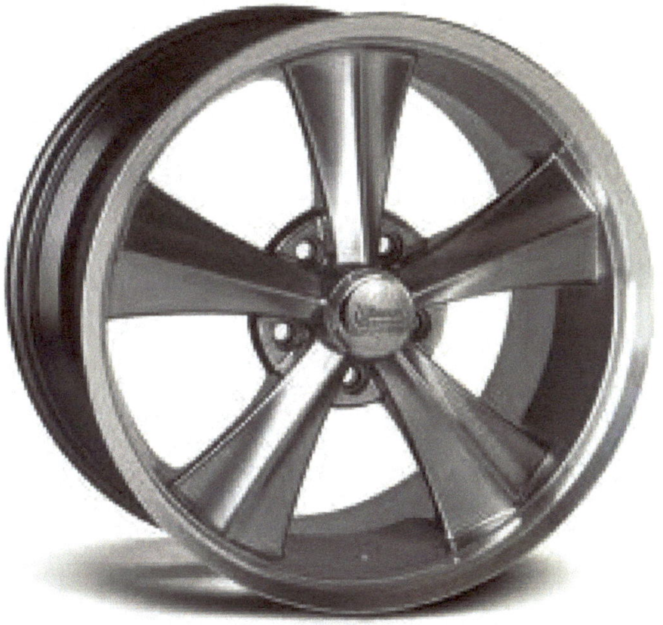

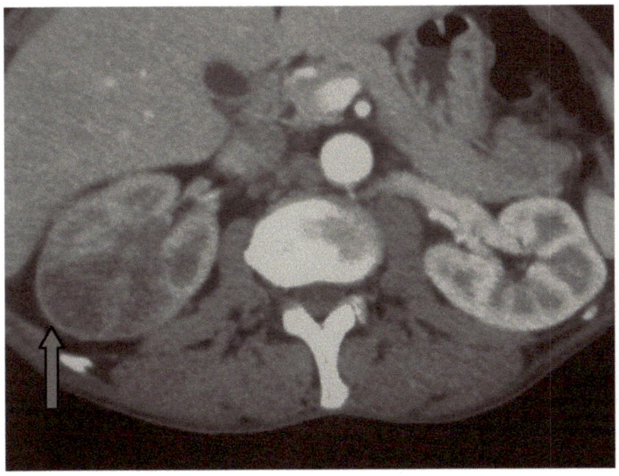

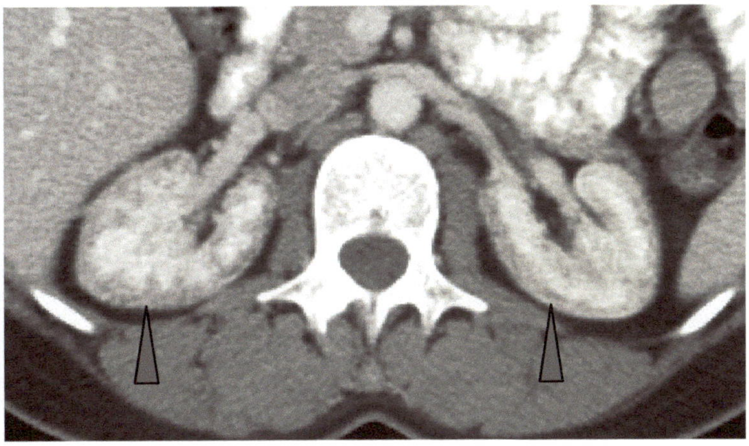

After IV enhancement, zones of renal infarction look like wedge-shaped low-density areas. Capsule and subcapsular kidney parenchyma is enhanced in many (but not all) patients due to collateral blood supply that forms the "*cortical rim*" sign (↑). This sign seldom occurs in pyelonephritis. For correct diagnosis the results must definitely correlate to clinical features.

In ischemic necrosis of the renal cortex, patients demonstrate enhancement of the medulla and capsule separated by a zone of cortical necrosis of low density forming the "*reversed rim*" sign (Δ). Up to 50 % of such cases refer to pregnancy complications and also shock and sepsis.

A. Yudin, *Metaphorical Signs in Computed Tomography of Chest and Abdomen*,
DOI 10.1007/978-3-319-04013-4_70, © Springer International Publishing Switzerland 2014

String of Beads Sign or String of Pearls Sign

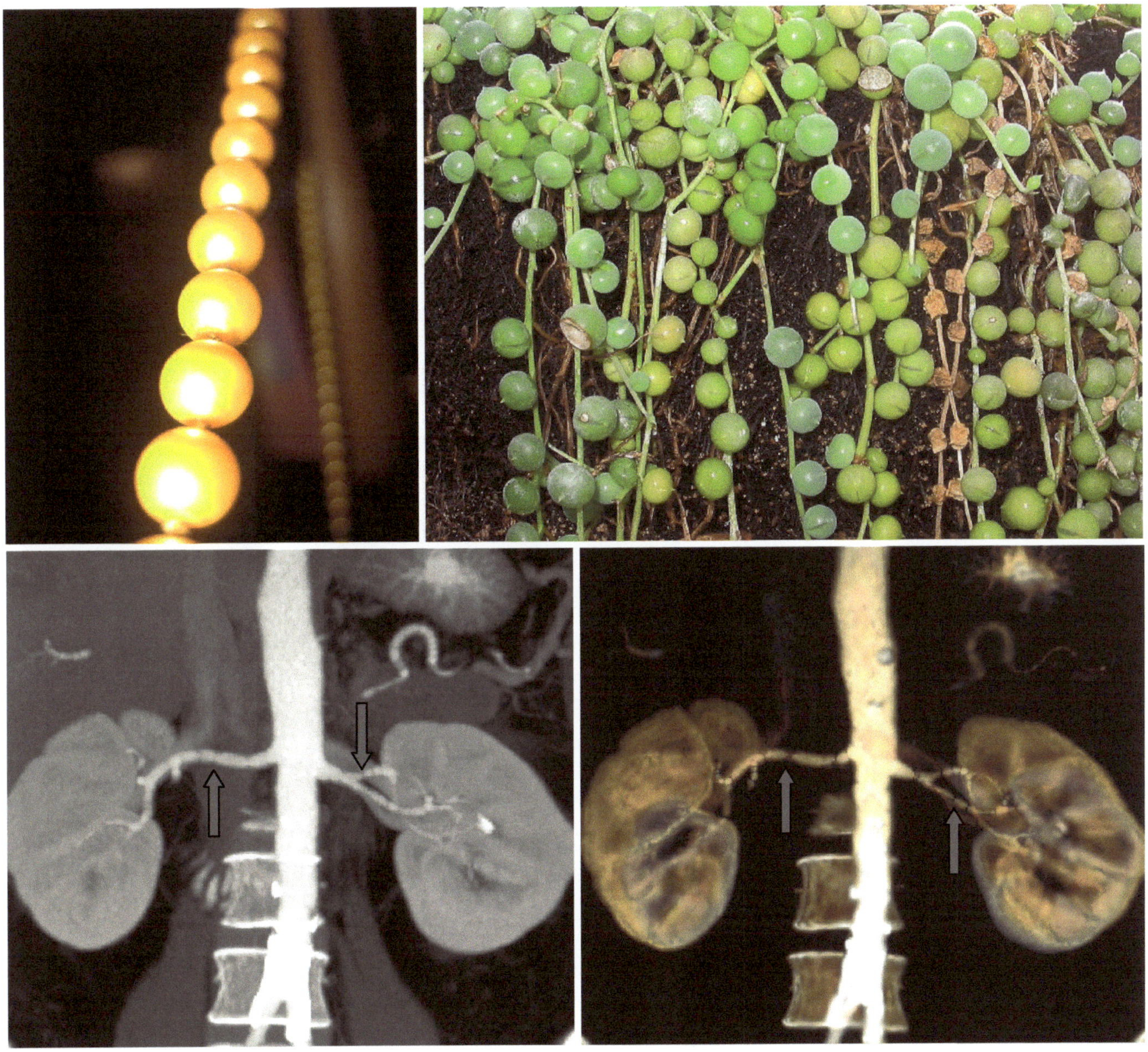

Fibromuscular dysplasia is the second in frequency disease causing renal artery stenoses. It is the most common cause of secondary arterial hypertension in young patients. After CT angiography beaded narrowings mainly of middle and distal segments of renal arteries may be found forming the "*string of beads*" sign or the "*string of pearls*" sign (↑).

A. Yudin, *Metaphorical Signs in Computed Tomography of Chest and Abdomen*,
DOI 10.1007/978-3-319-04013-4_71, © Springer International Publishing Switzerland 2014

Soft Tissue Rim Sign and Comet Sign

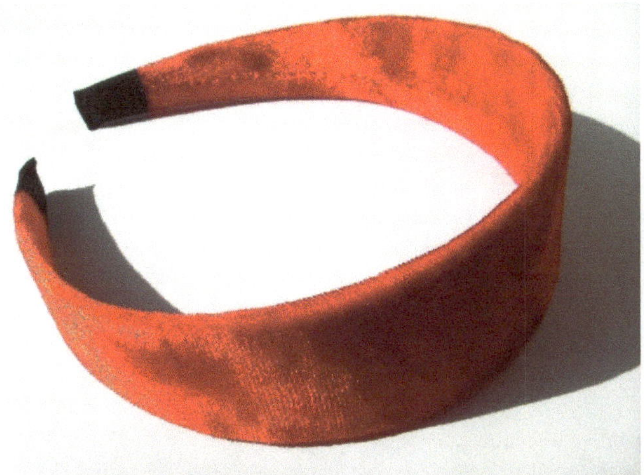

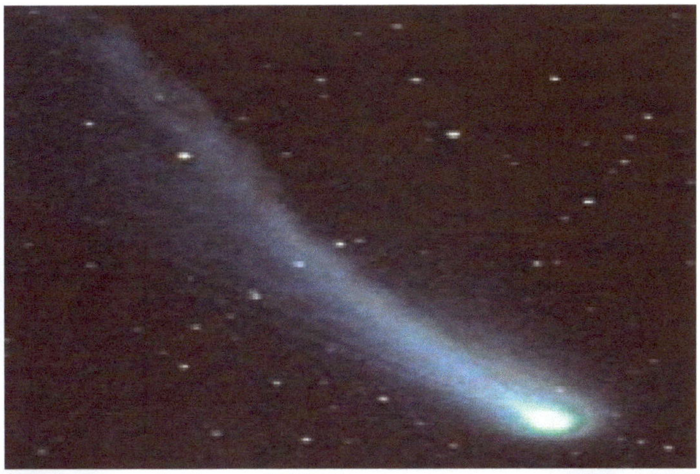

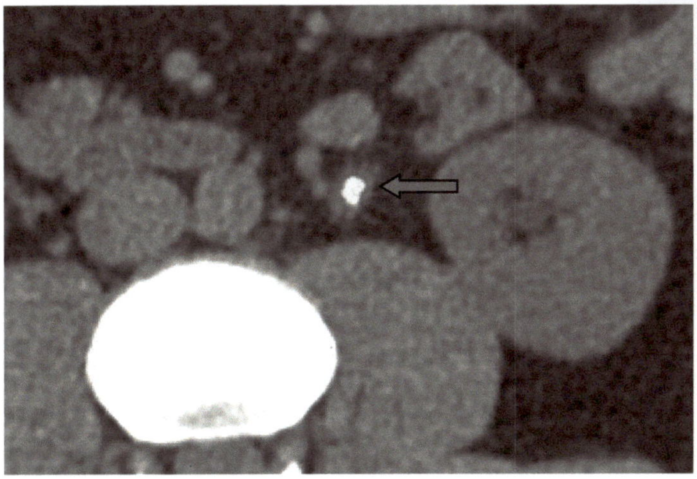

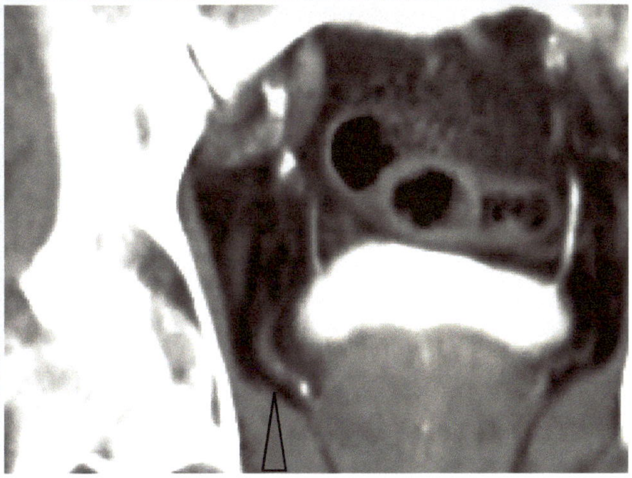

Concrements in the ureter cause edema and probably tissue inflammation that leads to wall thickening and periureteral stranding in ambient adipose tissue with formation of the "*soft tissue rim*" sign (↑). This sign is never noted around phleboliths.

A curved line of a vein and phlebolith (always without the rim of soft tissue) visible in the tomographic plane can form the "*comet*" sign (Δ). Thin collimation of X-rays and multiplanar reconstructions confidently help to determine the relationship of a ureter and a concrement as well as a vein and a phlebolith.

A. Yudin, *Metaphorical Signs in Computed Tomography of Chest and Abdomen*,
DOI 10.1007/978-3-319-04013-4_72, © Springer International Publishing Switzerland 2014

Whirlpool, Whirl, Swirl, and Whirling Sign

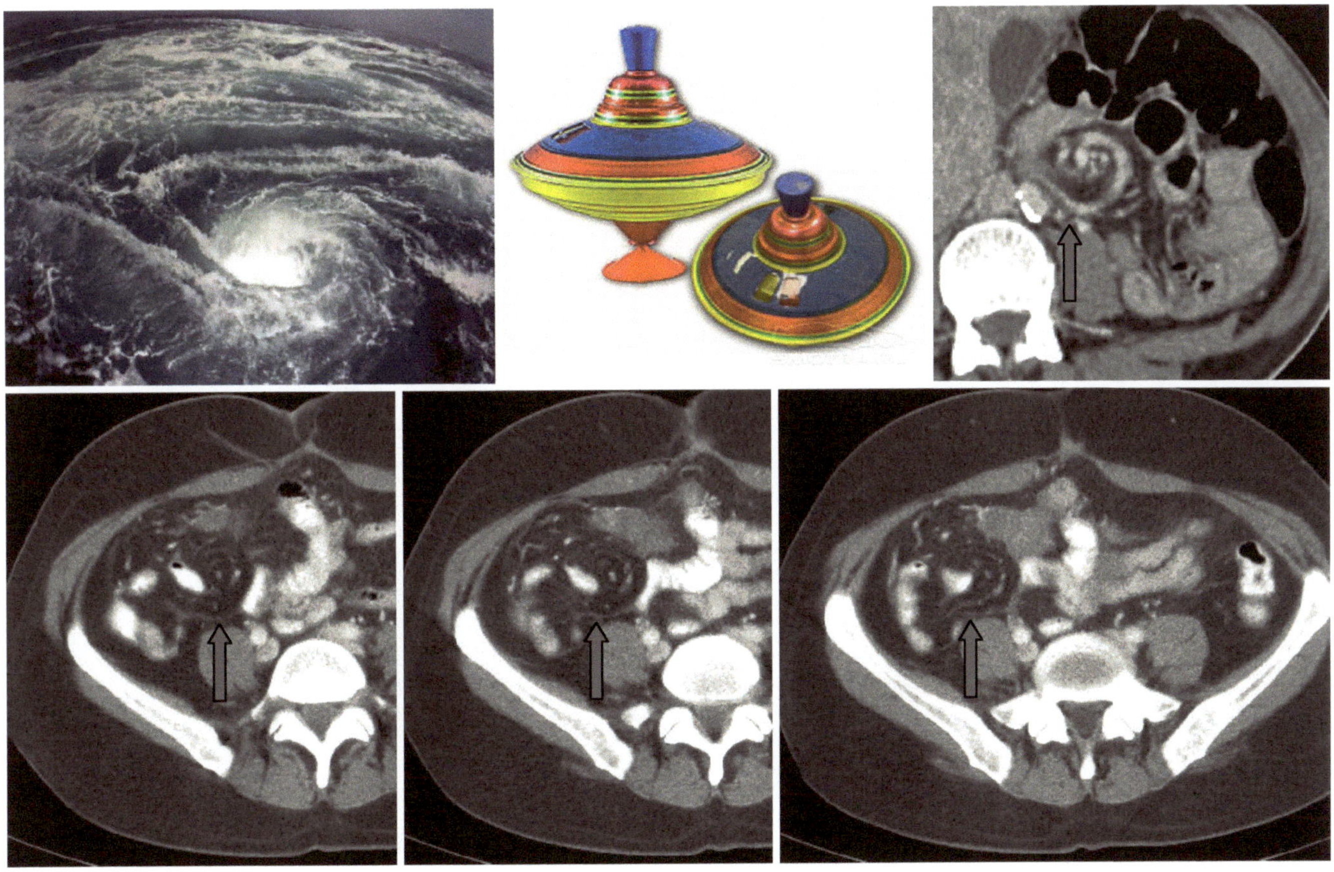

The "*whirlpool*" sign (also known as the "*whirl*", "*swirl*," and "*whirling*" sign) can be found in patients with small bowel volvulus (usually as a complication of bowel malrotation). On axial tomograms rotation of the intestine, mesentery, and superior mesenteric vein occurs around the superior mesenteric artery in a counterclockwise direction (↑). Curved mesenteric vessels form the image of a whirlpool. This sign can be seen also at the cecal and sigmoid volvulus.

Most distinctly the rotation is distinguished when studying cine CT scans.

A. Yudin, *Metaphorical Signs in Computed Tomography of Chest and Abdomen*,
DOI 10.1007/978-3-319-04013-4_73, © Springer International Publishing Switzerland 2014

Comb Sign

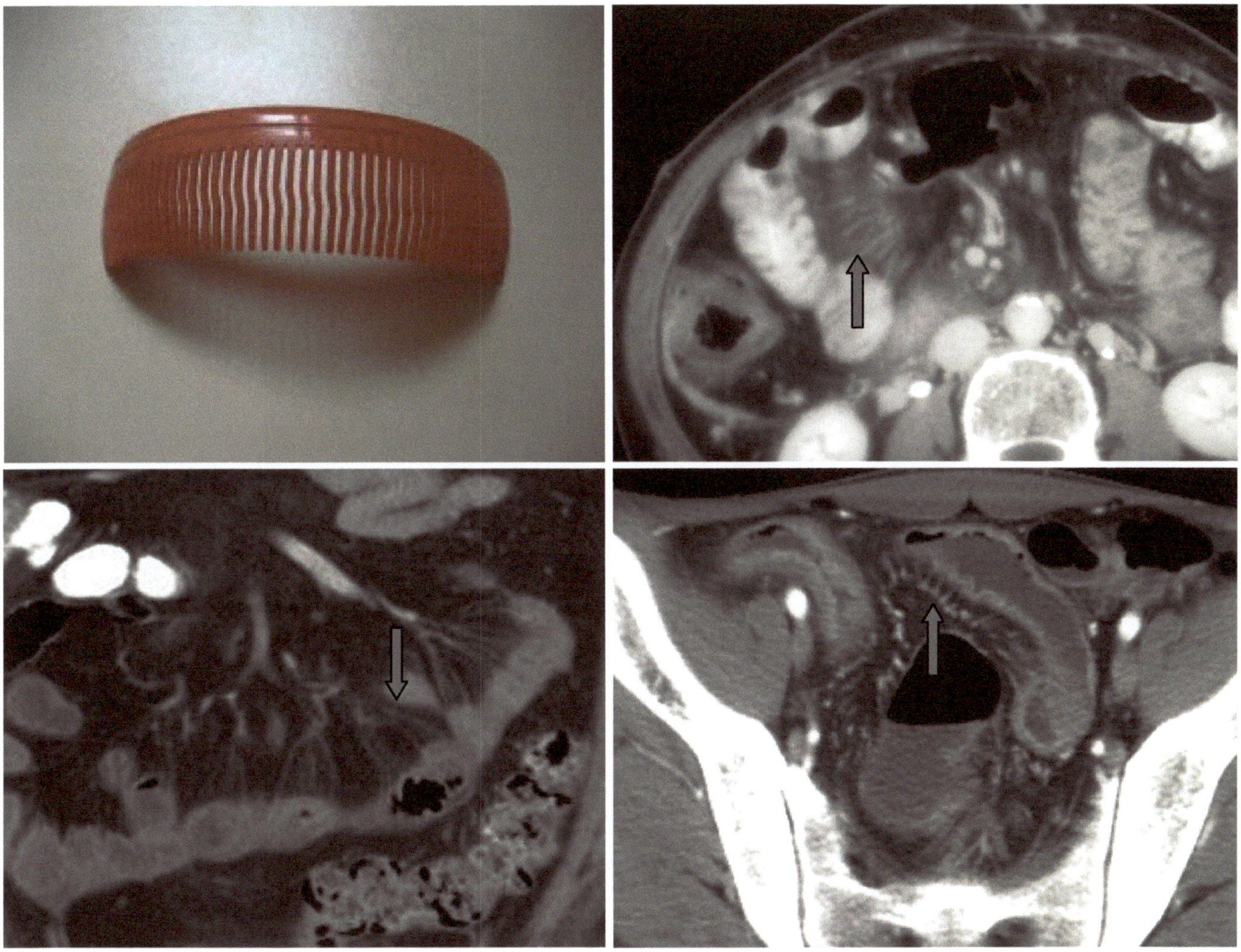

The increases in mesenteric blood flow and perivascular inflammatory infiltration form the image of linear structures near the bowel on the side of the mesentery forming the "*comb*" sign (↑). This sign is most often seen in Crohn disease and in ulcerative colitis. In any case it is the sign of active inflammatory process.

A. Yudin, *Metaphorical Signs in Computed Tomography of Chest and Abdomen*,
DOI 10.1007/978-3-319-04013-4_74, © Springer International Publishing Switzerland 2014

Stratified Attenuation, Double Halo Sign, and Target Sign

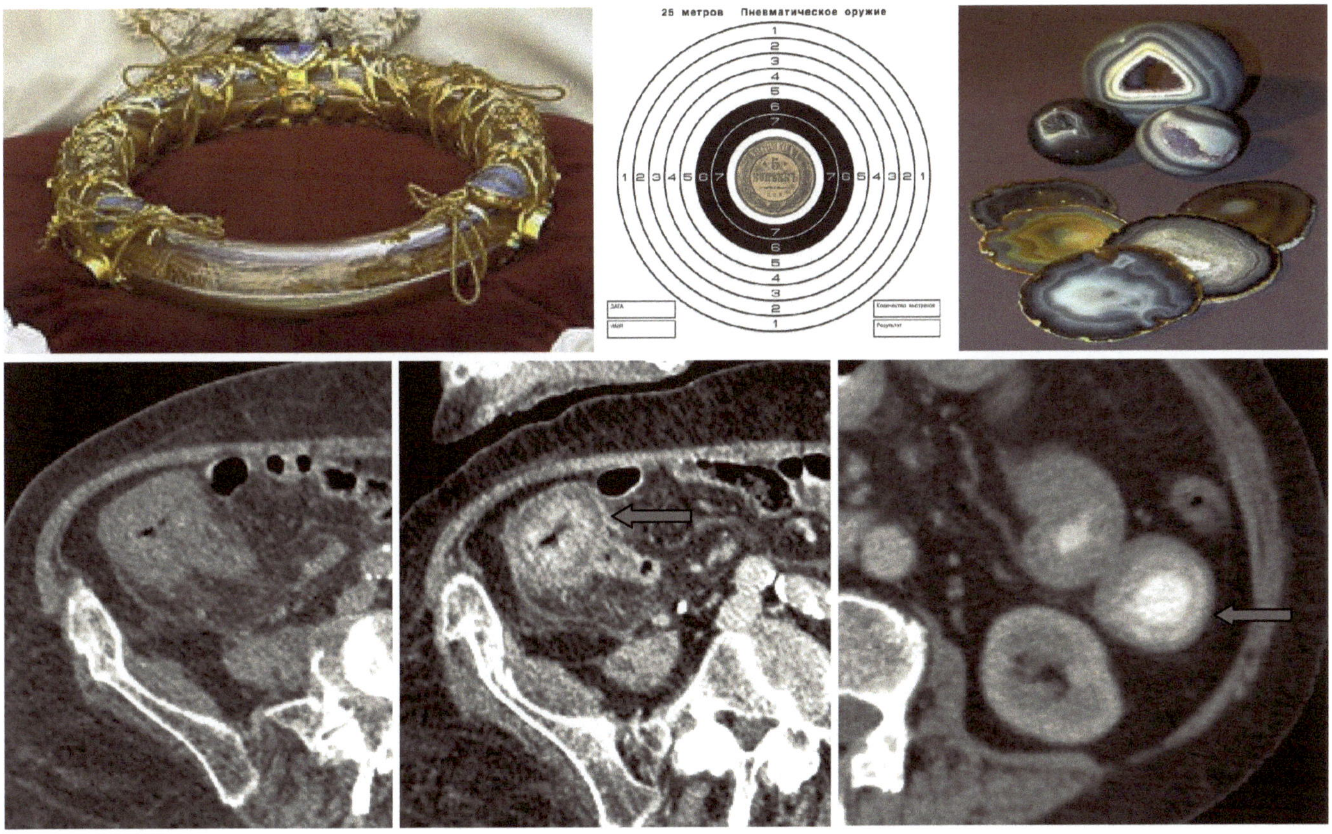

Stratified attenuation of bowel segments may take the form of a double circlet (with internal layer of low density and external layer of high density) forming the "*double halo*" sign or a target (with internal and external layers of high density and middle zone of low density) forming the "*target*" sign (↑). These signs usually reflect acute inflammation or ischemia. The layers with high density mean hyperemia and the layers with low density mean edema.

A. Yudin, *Metaphorical Signs in Computed Tomography of Chest and Abdomen*,
DOI 10.1007/978-3-319-04013-4_75, © Springer International Publishing Switzerland 2014

Target Sign, Sausage-Shaped Mass, and Reniform or Kidney-Shaped Bowel

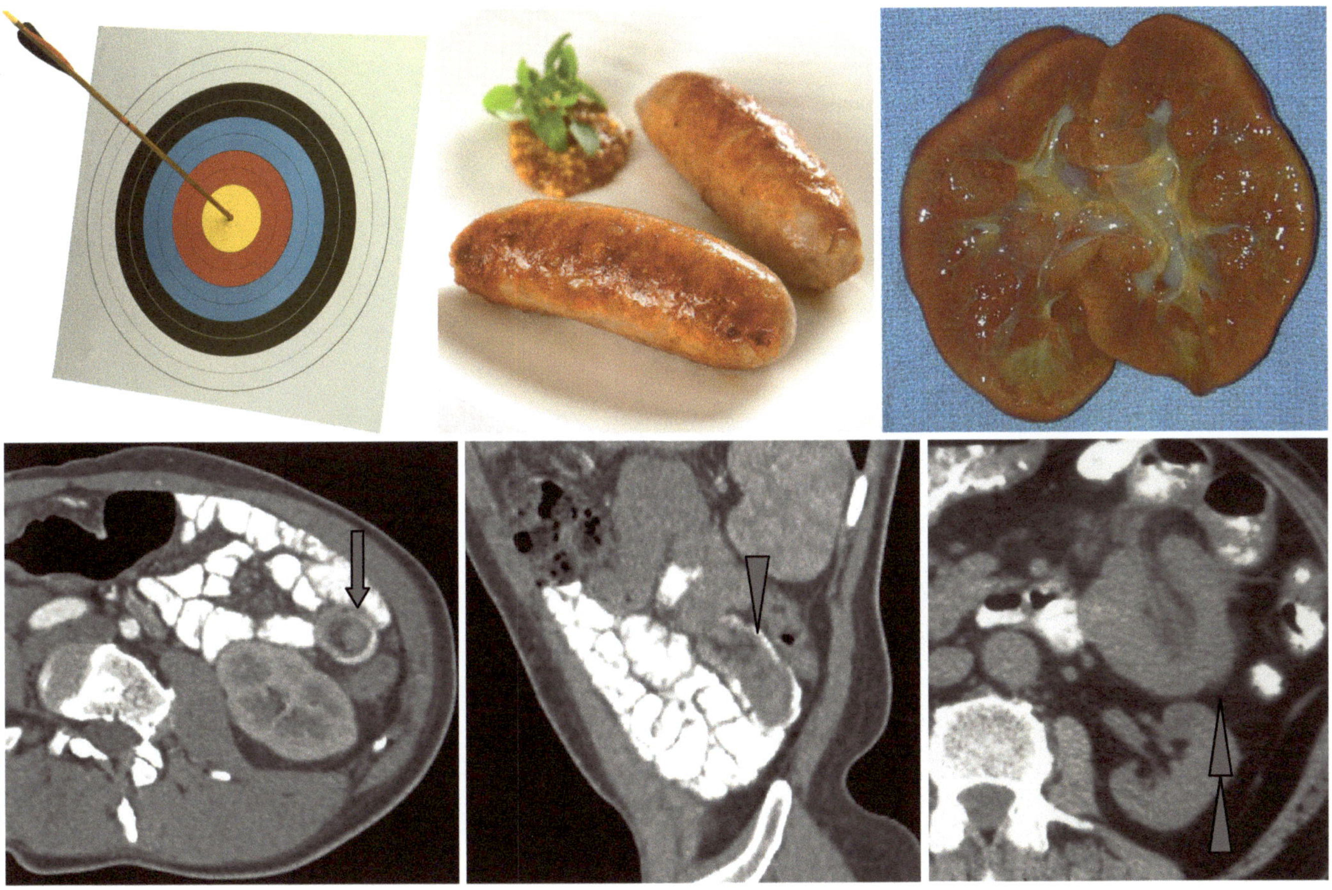

Invagination is the prolapse of the intestine loop together with a part of the mesentery inside the neighboring segment of the bowel. Three variants of bowel image on tomograms are described with invaginations:

1. Soft tissue formation in the bowel with eccentric location of the mesentery with fatty density – the "*target*" sign (↑)
2. *Sausage-shaped mass* (Δ) with alternating sites of low and high density of the bowel wall, mesentery, fluid, gas, and contrast medium
3. *Reniform* or *kidney-shaped bowel* (►►) with thickened bowel walls and edematous mesentery

The first variant refers to initial manifestations with a minimal degree of obstruction, but the second and the third ones refer to late changes with ileus and ischemia.

A. Yudin, *Metaphorical Signs in Computed Tomography of Chest and Abdomen*,
DOI 10.1007/978-3-319-04013-4_76, © Springer International Publishing Switzerland 2014

Fat Halo Sign

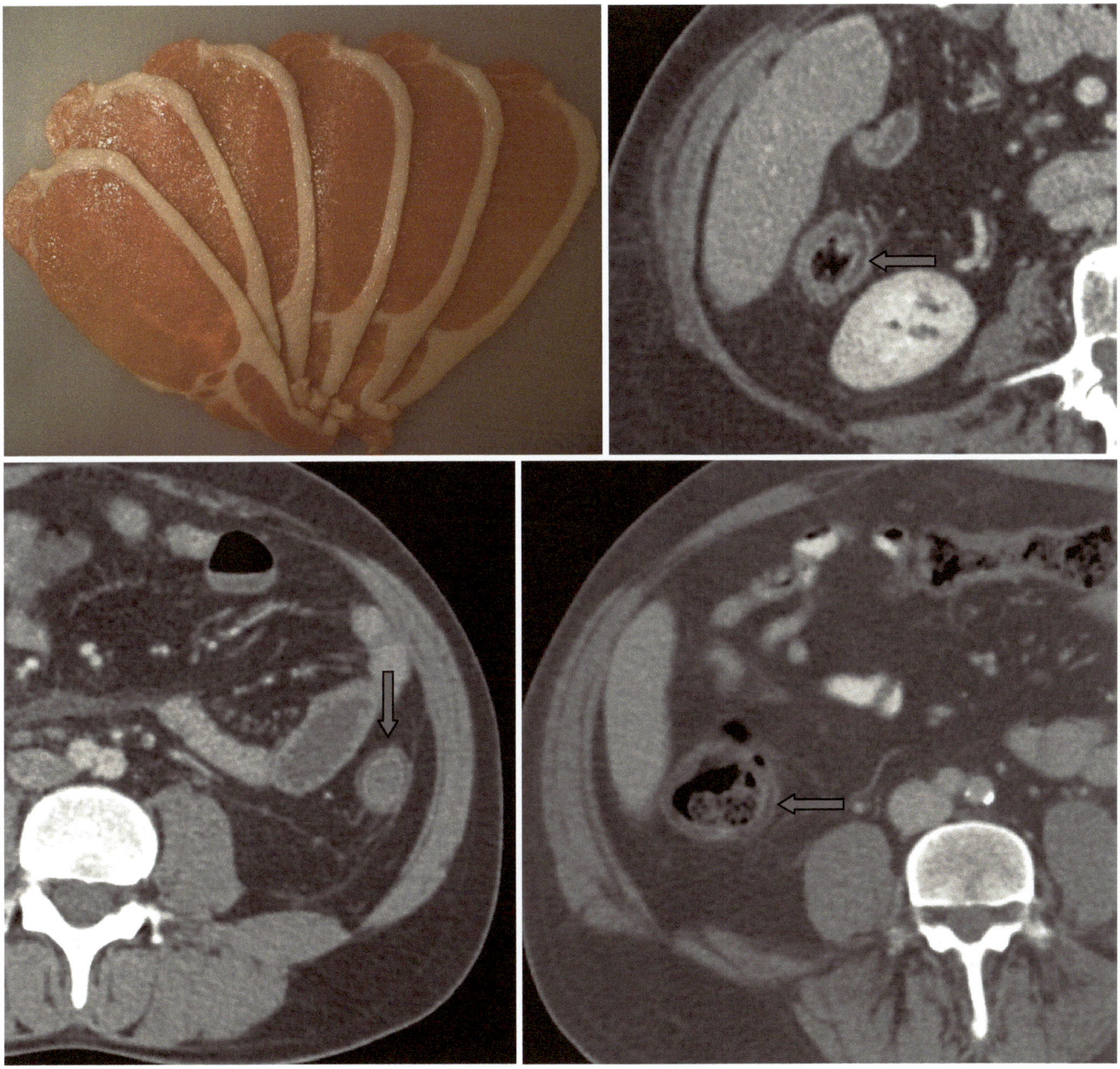

Fatty infiltration of the submucosal bowel layer – the "*fat halo*" sign (↑) – can be regarded as specific for inflammatory bowel diseases (Crohn disease, ulcerative colitis), but unlike the "double halo" sign and the "target" sign, it indicates the chronic stage of disease.

A. Yudin, *Metaphorical Signs in Computed Tomography of Chest and Abdomen*,
DOI 10.1007/978-3-319-04013-4_77, © Springer International Publishing Switzerland 2014

Accordion Sign

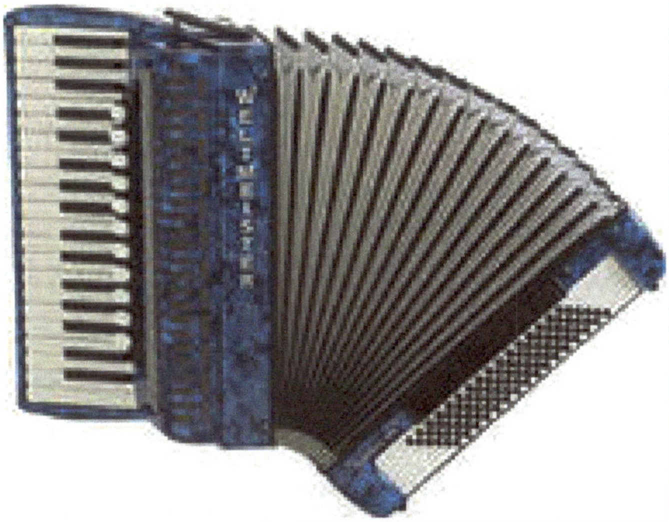

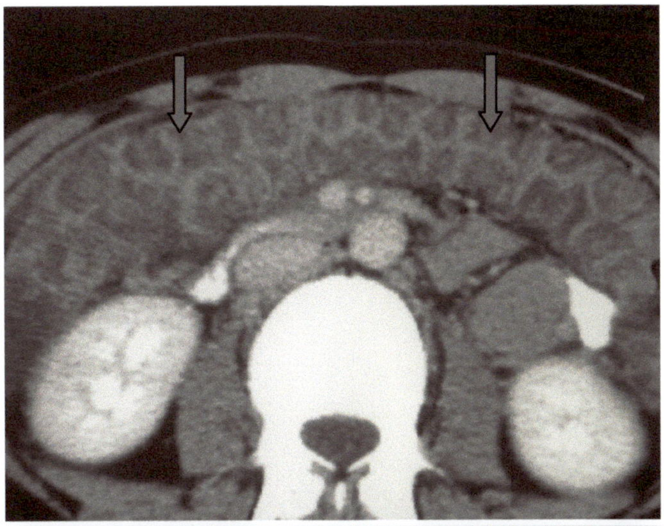

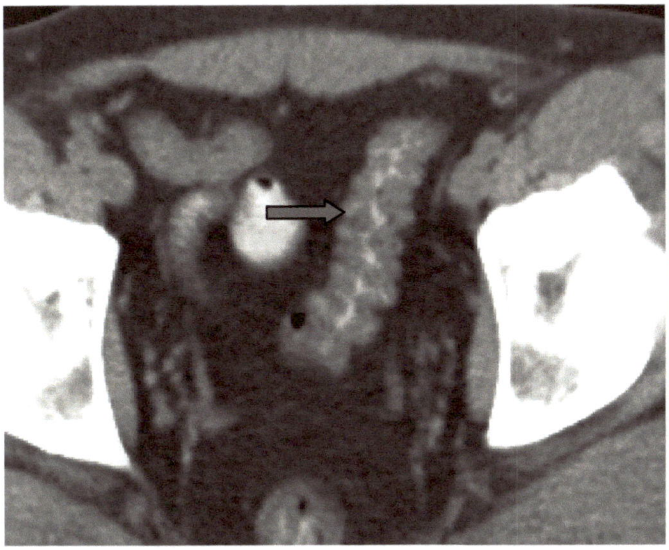

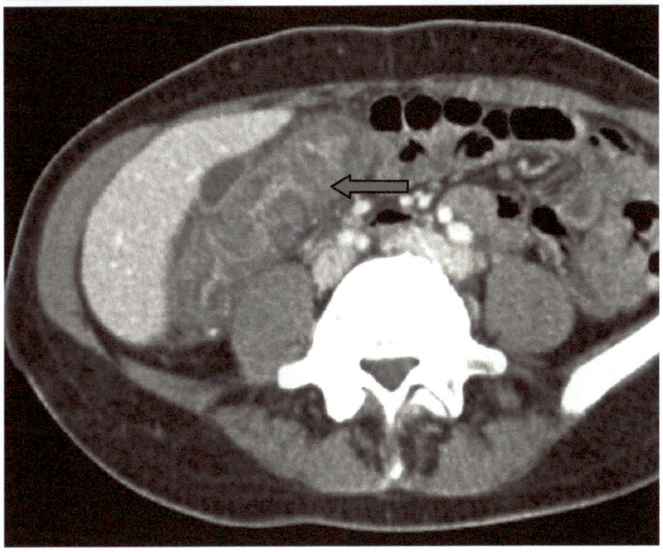

The increased enhancement of mucosa and submucosal edema of low density may form the "*accordion*" sign (↑) characteristic of pseudomembranous colitis. This sign also can be seen in other inflammatory processes, massive blood loss ("shock" bowel), mesentery thrombosis, edema, and hypoalbuminemia. It is necessary to correlate CT features to clinical data.

A. Yudin, *Metaphorical Signs in Computed Tomography of Chest and Abdomen*,
DOI 10.1007/978-3-319-04013-4_78, © Springer International Publishing Switzerland 2014

Rim Enhancement or Target Sign

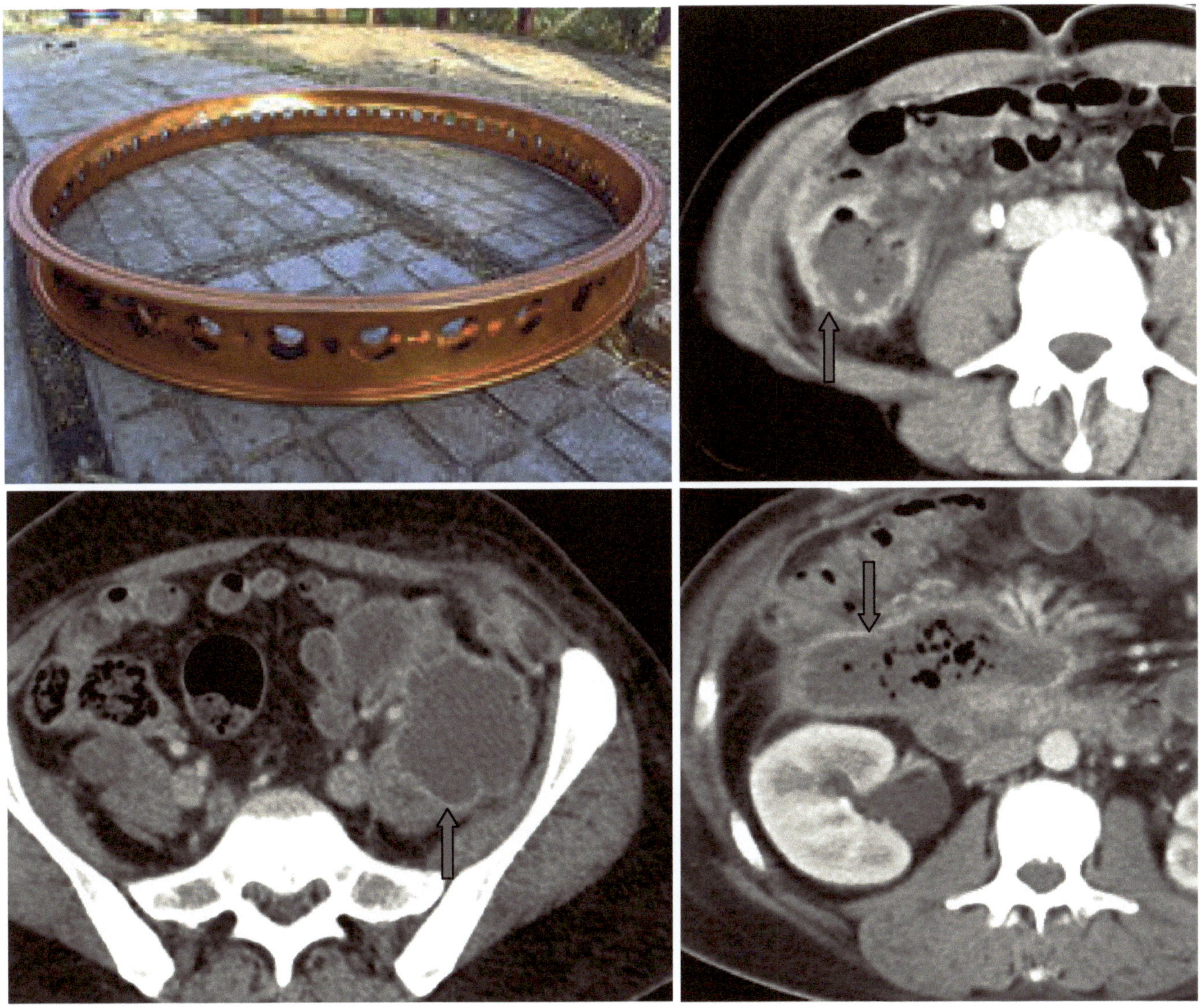

An abdominal abscess represents a collection of pus limited to a fibrocapillary "capsule." After IV enhancement, the capsule intensively accumulates the contrast agent but internal contents keep low density – the "*rim enhancement*" or the "*target*" sign (↑). In 50 % of patients, gas bubbles in the abscess can be observed. In 10 % of patients in an appendicular abscess, an appendicolith may be found which is better seen on native images.

A. Yudin, *Metaphorical Signs in Computed Tomography of Chest and Abdomen*,
DOI 10.1007/978-3-319-04013-4_79, © Springer International Publishing Switzerland 2014

Soap Bubble Appearance and Small Bowel Feces Sign

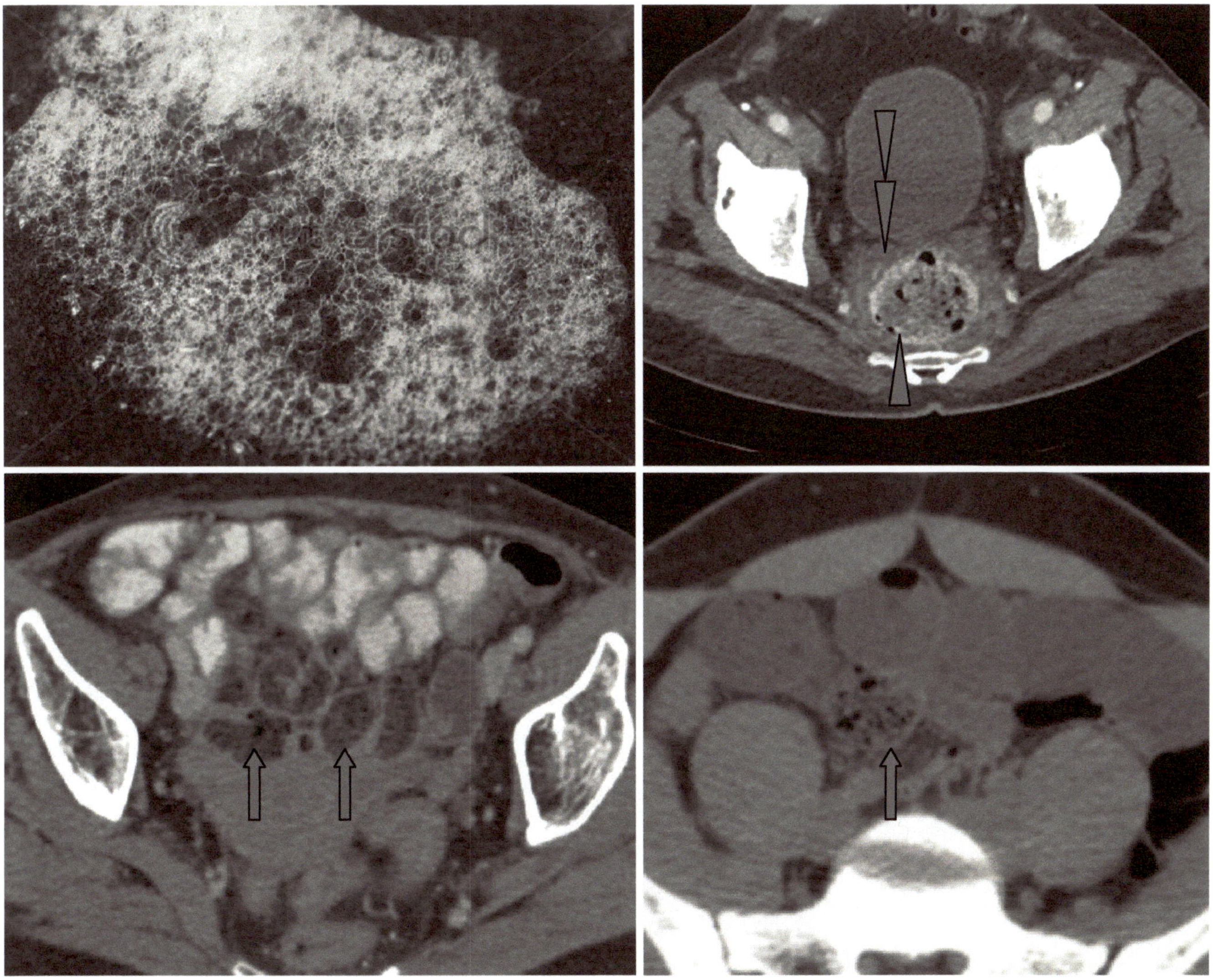

On tomograms colonic fecal masses look like lather due to a considerable amount of gas bubbles – *soap bubble appearance* (Δ). It is possible to find a colonic wall thickening and increased density of fatty tissue due to inflammation in chronic constipations around such a fecaloma. This set of features suggests the presence of a fecal ulcer (stercoral ulceration) as a necrosis caused by the pressure on the bowel wall (►►).

The presence of a substrate similar to colonic fecal masses in the small intestine – the "*small bowel feces*" sign (↑) – first of all creates suspicion of subacute or partial small bowel obstruction. Such changes can also be found out in small bowel dysfunction (metabolic or infectious diseases).

A. Yudin, *Metaphorical Signs in Computed Tomography of Chest and Abdomen*,
DOI 10.1007/978-3-319-04013-4_80,

Ring Sign

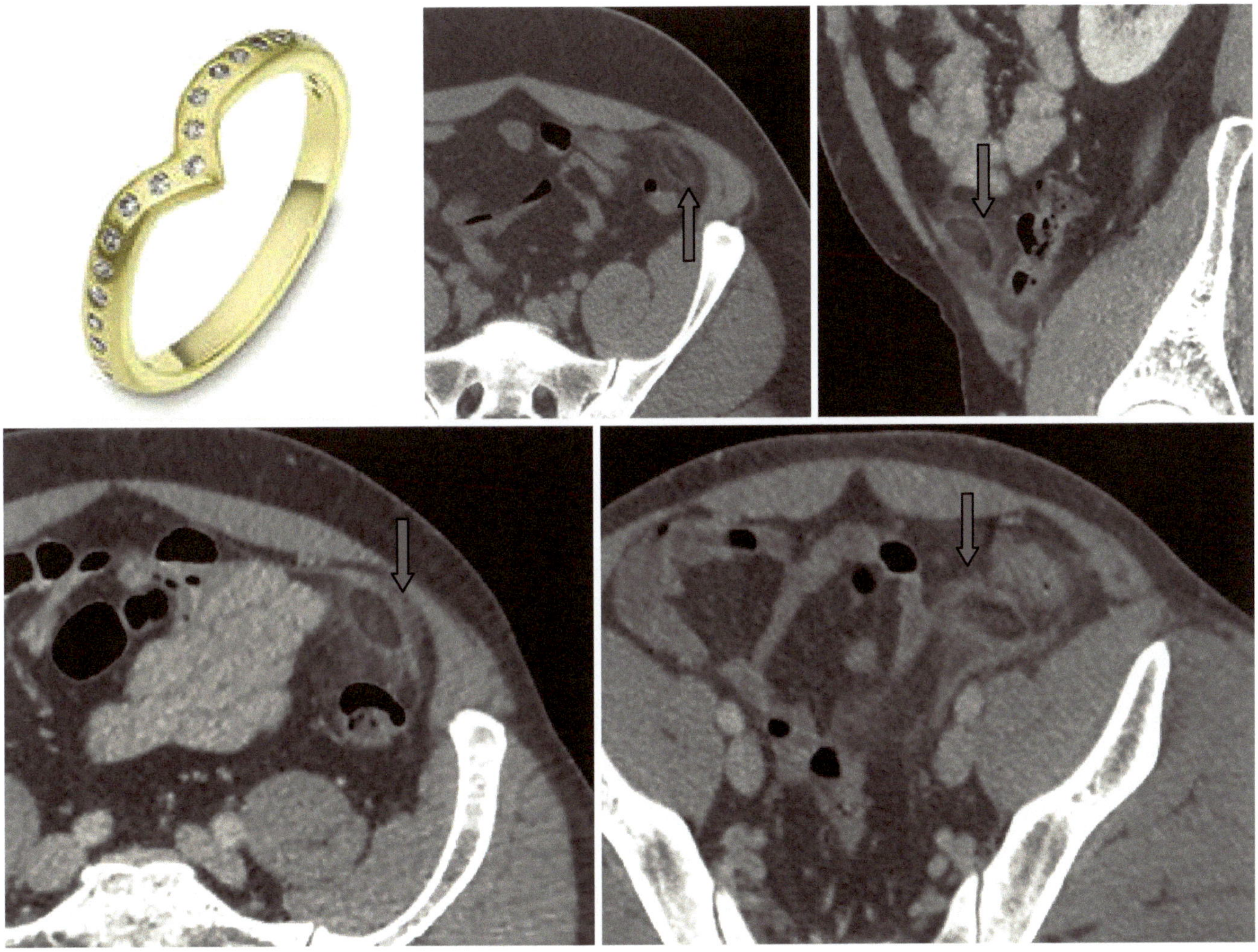

Acute inflammation or infarct of a mesenteric appendage (epiploic appendagitis) can be detected on tomograms as a structure of oval or irregular form containing fatty tissue and surrounded by a thin hyperdense ring – the "*ring*" sign (↑). Signs of inflammation of surrounding fat can also be visible. A dense "point" may be seen in the center representing a thrombosed vein.

A. Yudin, *Metaphorical Signs in Computed Tomography of Chest and Abdomen*,
DOI 10.1007/978-3-319-04013-4_81, © Springer International Publishing Switzerland 2014

Omental Cake Sign

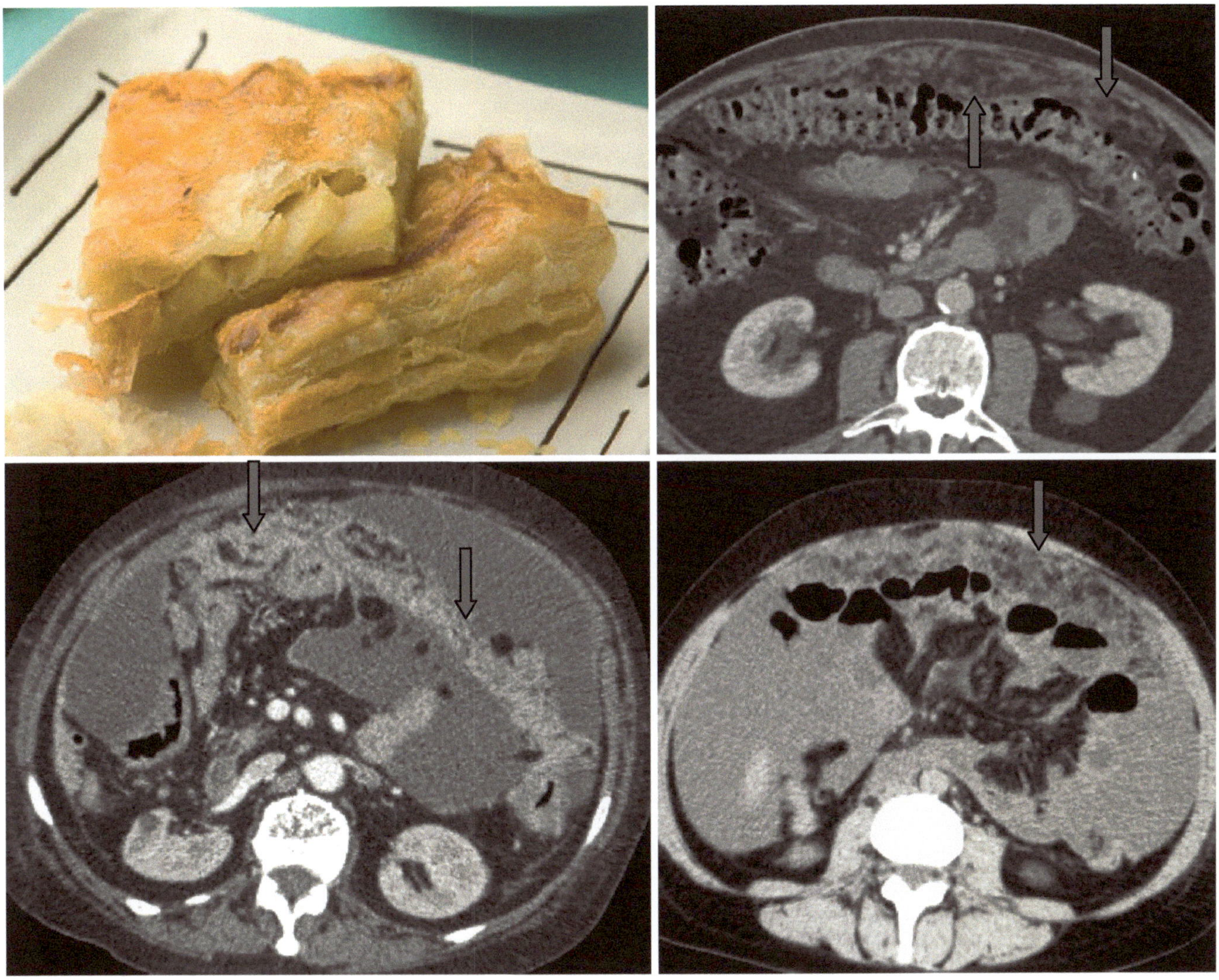

The pathologically thickened and infiltrated omentum forms the "*omental cake*" sign on tomograms (↑). After IV injection of contrast agent, the omentum enhances irregularly and shows the cellular structure imitating a layer cake. The most frequent causes for infiltration of the large omentum are metastases from carcinomas of the ovaries, stomach, and colon. Also similar images of omental infiltration can be found in tuberculous peritonitis and, extremely seldom, in primary tumors of the large omentum (mesothelioma in particular).

A. Yudin, *Metaphorical Signs in Computed Tomography of Chest and Abdomen*,
DOI 10.1007/978-3-319-04013-4_82, © Springer International Publishing Switzerland 2014

Sandwich Sign

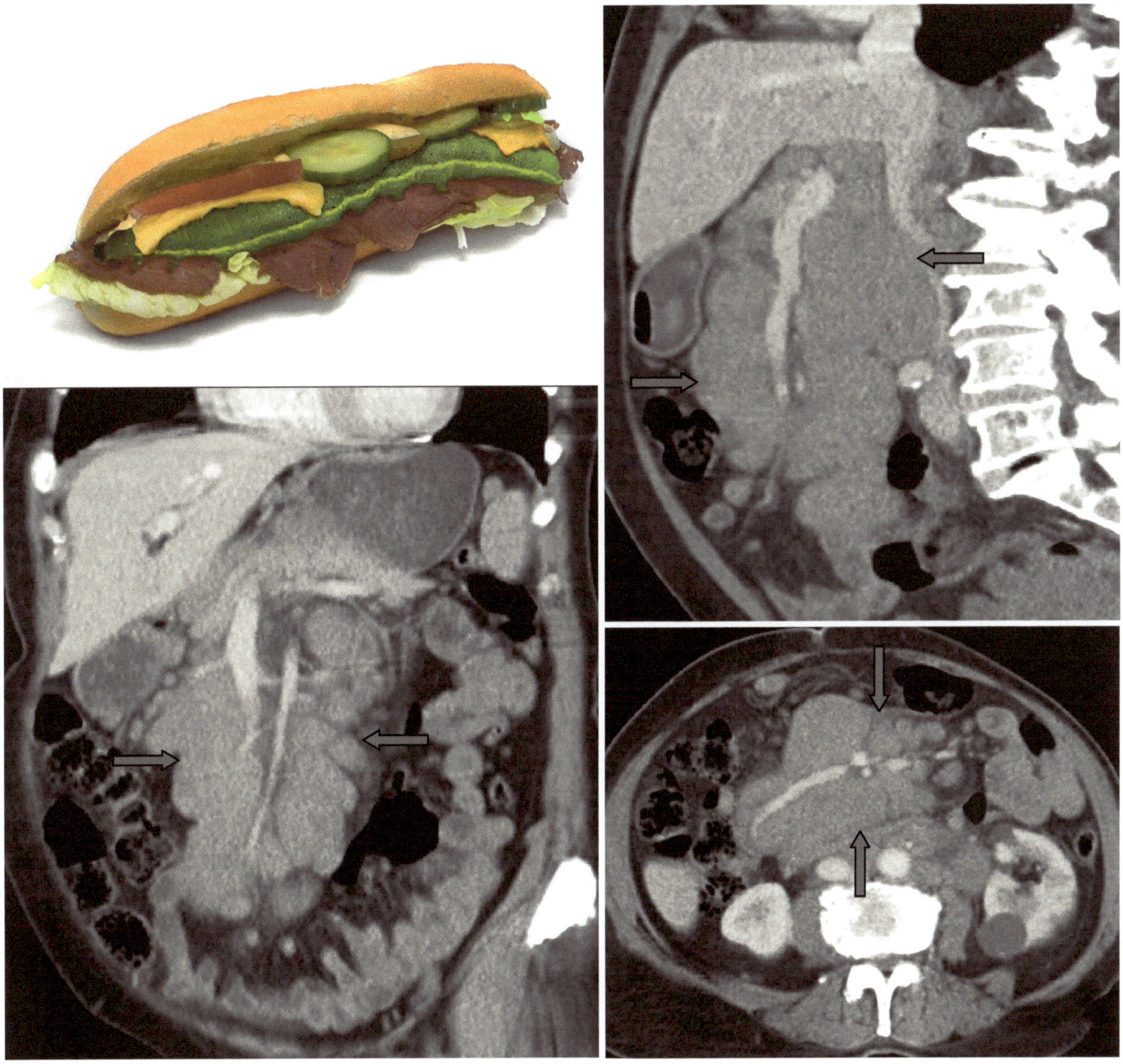

The "*sandwich*" sign (↑) is formed in lymphomas of the mesentery when the enlarged lymph nodes surround the enhanced mesenteric vessels. Damage to the mesenteric lymph nodes occurs in non-Hodgkin's lymphomas (>50 %), whereas in Hodgkin's lymphoma, it is seen in not more than 5 % of the surveyed.

A. Yudin, *Metaphorical Signs in Computed Tomography of Chest and Abdomen*,
DOI 10.1007/978-3-319-04013-4_83, © Springer International Publishing Switzerland 2014

Misty Mesentery Sign and Fat Halo Sign

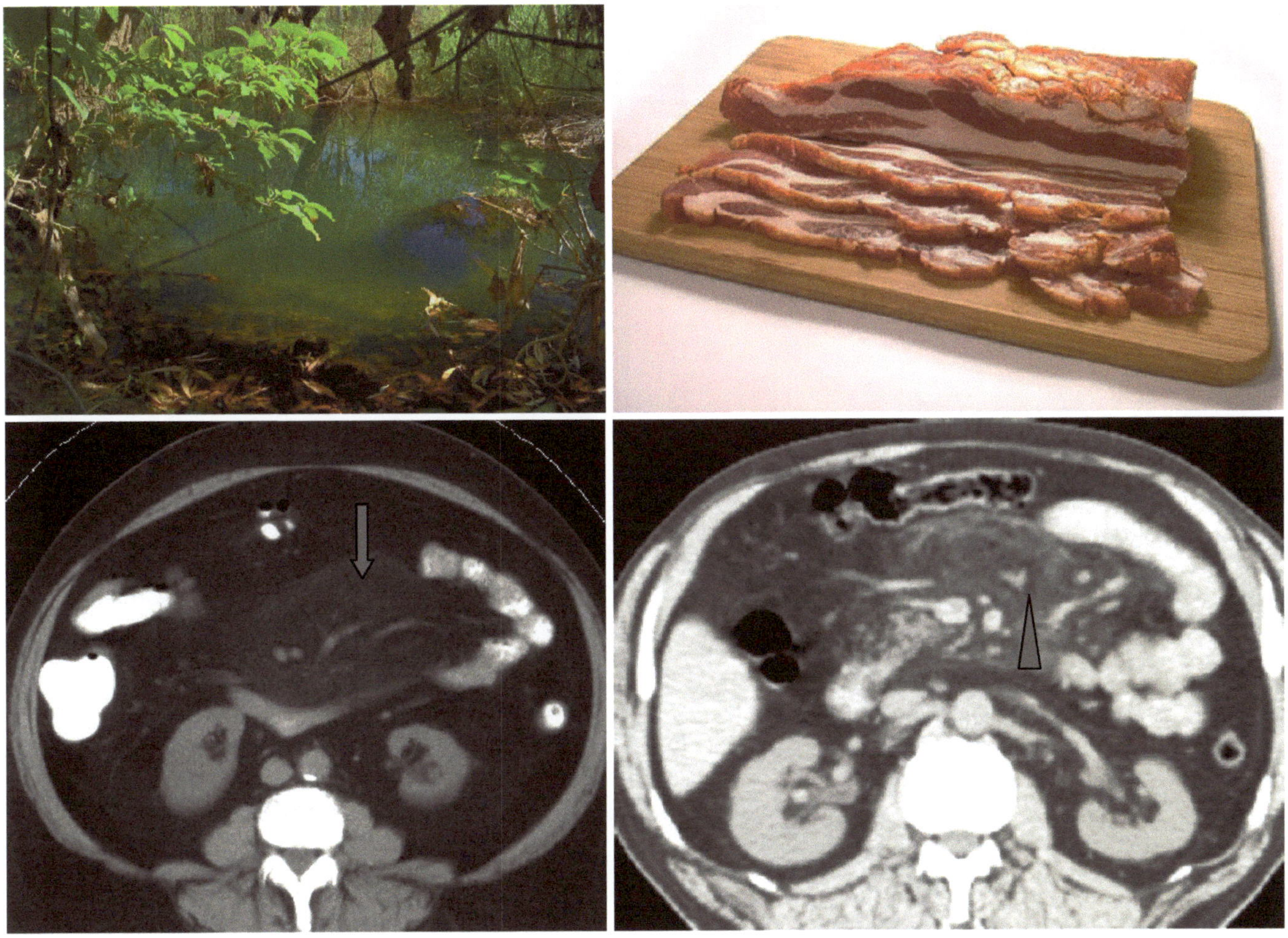

Any inflammatory and proliferative process involving mesenteric tissues leads to increase in the density of the fatty tissue – the "*misty mesentery*" sign (↑). The most probable idiopathic variant is mesenteric panniculitis (sclerosing mesenteritis). In addition to the "misty mesentery," the specific feature of mesenteric panniculitis must be defined as the rim of normal fatty density around mesenteric vessels – the "*fat halo*" sign (Δ). Unlike liposarcomas the mass effect is absent. In differential diagnostics in the presence of the "misty mesentery" sign, it is necessary to consider hypoalbuminemia, cirrhosis, lymphedema, pancreatitis, tuberculosis, bleeding, non-Hodgkin's lymphoma, cholelithiasis, peptic ulcer and carcinoma of the stomach, blunt abdominal trauma, autoimmune diseases, and so forth.

A. Yudin, *Metaphorical Signs in Computed Tomography of Chest and Abdomen*,
DOI 10.1007/978-3-319-04013-4_84,

Dirty Fat Sign

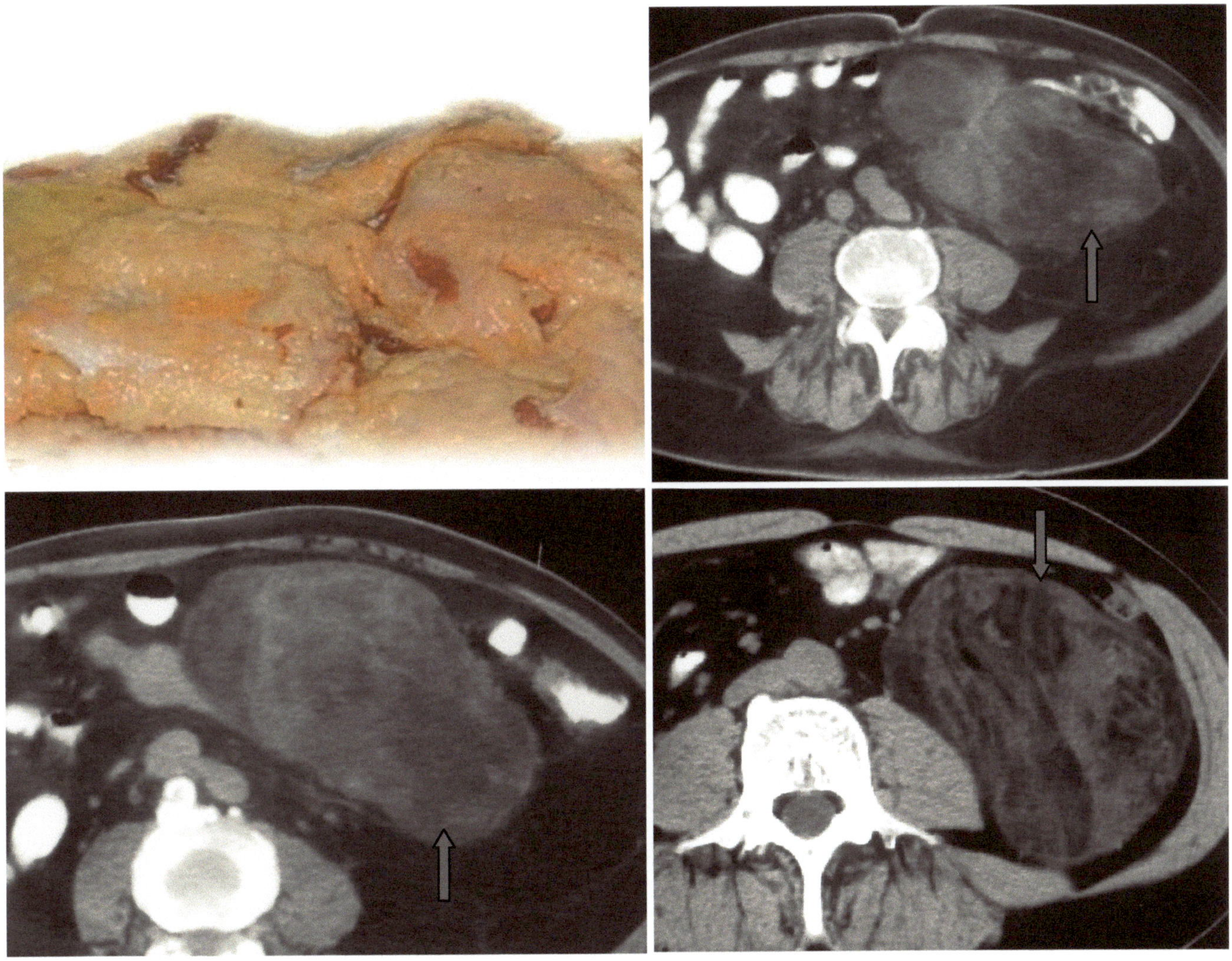

Liposarcomas of the retroperitoneal space are characterized by three variants of images on tomograms, based on the amount of fat in different parts of the tumor.

1. The mixed variant (mixed pattern) – sites of a fatty tissue alternate with soft tissue zones and vessels – the "*dirty fat*" sign (↑). It is the most frequent pattern.
2. The soft tissue variant (solid pattern) – mass with density higher than +20HU, nonuniform (mainly myxoid tissue).
3. Pseudocystic variant (pseudocystic pattern) – mass of homogeneous density from −20 HU to +20 HU.

   In liposarcomas, the "claw or beak" sign is always absent.

A. Yudin, *Metaphorical Signs in Computed Tomography of Chest and Abdomen*,
DOI 10.1007/978-3-319-04013-4_85, © Springer International Publishing Switzerland 2014

Hematocrit Sign

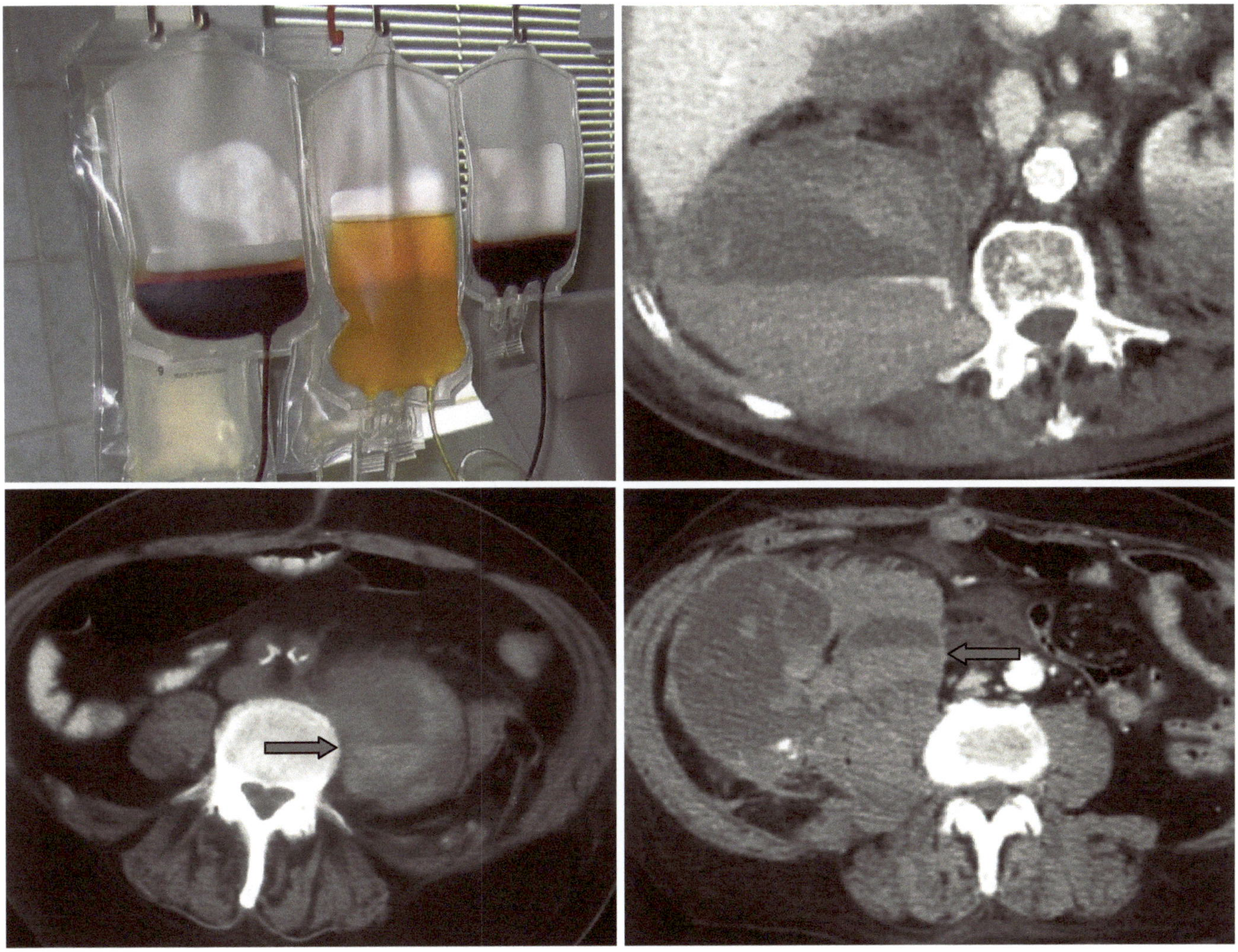

Coagulopathic retroperitoneal hemorrhages become apparent as the zones of high density in the retroperitoneal space, muscles, and tissues. A horizontal level between blood with high density and tissues is usually found, forming the "*hematocrit*" sign (↑). Most of the so-called retroperitoneal bleedings form in the posterior abdominal wall muscles. The most common causes for bleedings include anticoagulant therapy and coagulopathy. After IV enhancement sites of various shapes with the density corresponding to the enhanced blood can be identified in active bleeding.

A. Yudin, *Metaphorical Signs in Computed Tomography of Chest and Abdomen*,
DOI 10.1007/978-3-319-04013-4_86, © Springer International Publishing Switzerland 2014

Recommended Literature

Algın O, Gökalp G, Topal U (2011) Signs in chest imaging. Diagn Interv Radiol 17:18–29

Baldwin M, Genant J, Braver J et al (2011) Classic signs in gastrointestinal radiology. Part 1. Appl Radiol 12:22–27

Baldwin M, Genant J, Braver J et al (2012) Classic signs in gastrointestinal radiology. Part 2. Appl Radiol 1:29–35

Dyer RB, Chen MY, Zagoria RJ (2004) Classic signs in uroradiology. Radiographics 24:S247–S280

Eisenberg RL (1984) Atlas of signs in radiology. Philadelphia: J.B. Lippincott, p 505

http://www.appliedradiology.com/Article.aspx?id=27386&terms=Classic+signs+in+gastrointestinal+radiology

http://en.wikipedia.org/wiki/Category:Radiologic_signs

http://findebookee.com/r/radiological-signs

Marshall GB, Farnquist BA, MacGregor JH et al (2006) Signs in thoracic imaging. J Thorac Imaging 21:76–90

Mehboob H, Al Damegh S (2007) Food signs in radiology. Int J Health Sci 1:168–178

Mulligan ME (1996) Classic radiologic signs: an atlas and history. New York, NY: Parthenon, p 208

Strang JG, Dogra VS (2006) Body CT secrets. Elsevier Science, New York, p 424

A. Yudin, *Metaphorical Signs in Computed Tomography of Chest and Abdomen*,
DOI 10.1007/978-3-319-04013-4, © Springer International Publishing Switzerland 2014

Index

A. Yudin, *Metaphorical Signs in Computed Tomography of Chest and Abdomen*,
DOI 10.1007/978-3-319-04013-4, © Springer International Publishing Switzerland 2014